How to Eat Well for Adults with ADHD

A Practical, Non-Diet Guide to Feeding Your Body & Mind When You Have ADHD

Rebecca King, MS, RDN

FAIR WINDS

Quarto.com

© 2025 Quarto Publishing Group USA Inc.

Text © 2025 Rebecca King

First Published in 2025 by Fair Winds Press, an imprint of The Quarto Group,
100 Cummings Center, Suite 265-D, Beverly, MA 01915, USA.
T (978) 282-9590 F (978) 283-2742

Fair Winds Press titles are also available at discount for retail, wholesale, promotional, and bulk purchase. For details, contact the Special Sales Manager by email at specialsales@quarto.com or by mail at The Quarto Group, Attn: Special Sales Manager, 100 Cummings Center, Suite 265-D, Beverly, MA 01915, USA.

29 28 27 26 25 1 2 3 4 5

ISBN: 978-0-7603-9208-9

Digital edition published in 2025
eISBN: 978-0-7603-9209-6

Library of Congress Cataloging-in-Publication Data available.

Cover Image: Abby Winkler (illustration) and Wendi Washington-Hunt (photography)
Design and Page Layout: Mattie Wells
Photography: Wendi Washington-Hunt, wwhfoodphotography.com
Illustration: Abby Winkler

Printed in China

Dedication

To my parents, Patty and Jim, my little sister, Ali, and my sweet puppy at heart, Lola, for all the unconditional love, support, and teaching me there is no "right way" to do things, including feeding yourself.

Disclaimer

I'd also like to take this moment to acknowledge that I am writing this book from the perspective of a cisgender, able-bodied bisexual, white woman with thin privilege. As someone who is bisexual and neurodivergent, I've experienced how having marginalized identities can make life more challenging. But I think it's really important to note I still have immense privileges that make navigating the world and my relationship with food easier. I don't have the lived experience of food insecurity or weight stigma, and I have so much empathy and compassion for anyone reading this who has.

Contents

Introduction ·································· 6

PART 1

THIS IS YOUR ADHD ON FOOD / 11

Chapter 1: How Does My ADHD Impact My Relationship with Food? ······ 12

Chapter 2: Intuitive Eating for ADHD ···················· 22

PART 2

HOW TO FEED YOURSELF WHEN YOU HAVE ADHD / 33

Chapter 3: Why Is It So Hard to Listen to My Body? ············· 34

Chapter 4: ADHDers Are Consistently Inconsistent . . . Including with Food ··· 47

Chapter 5: Why Am I Such an Emotional Eater? ··············· 58

Chapter 6: ADHD: The Food and Dopamine Connection ········· 70

Chapter 7: Gentle Nutrition for ADHD and Why It Matters ·········· 81

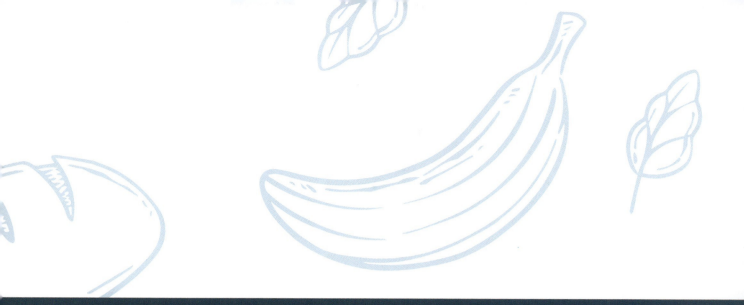

PART 3

LET'S GET COOKING! / 105

Chapter 8: Overcoming Overwhelm in the Kitchen ·································· 106

Chapter 9: Easy Non-Diet Recipes for Adults with ADHD ················· 128

Resources ·· 186
Acknowledgments ··· 187
About the Author ·· 188
Index ·· 189

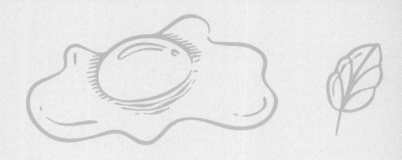

Introduction

As an adult ADHDer and registered dietitian, I know how complicated your relationship with food can be. I also know that shame can result when you struggle with feeding yourself nutritious foods.

ADHD impacts every part of an ADHDer's life, including their relationship with food. Often, I find the things society labels as "easy," like cooking, eating, sleeping, staying hydrated, cleaning, and moving regularly, are the very areas of life that ADHDers struggle with the most.

In an ideal world, when someone is diagnosed, they would be given a care team of providers to support them with managing their ADHD. They would have a doctor to manage meds, a therapist for emotional support, an ADHD coach to help with day-to-day strategies, a dietitian to support healthy nutrition, a trainer, an occupational therapist, and a peer-support group to provide connection and community. Unfortunately, this isn't the reality for most people. Hopefully this book will help with the food piece of the puzzle.

One of the most common statements I hear from ADHDers is **"It's not that I don't know what to do, it's that I don't know how to do it."** This leaves ADHDers feeling broken, incapable of being adults, stuck, and confused. If you feel like this, please know that you are not alone and I'm here to help you.

My Struggle with ADHD and Food

Like many other women who were diagnosed with ADHD later in life, I look back on my childhood and wonder how I wasn't diagnosed sooner. I was a hyperactive kid, so my mom kept me busy with gymnastics, ballet, swimming, and basketball. The basketball court was a sanctuary where my brain felt calm, and I learned the power of being able to hyperfocus.

I learned to mask my hyperactivity in class by chewing gum and my inability to pay attention by maintaining eye contact and nodding along with what my teachers were saying. Although I made good grades, I had to spend A LOT more time studying, using different study "tricks" than my peers, and getting a tutor so I didn't fail eighth-grade algebra and got a decent SAT score.

I struggled with regulating alertness, so as a kid I would stay up late at night pacing up and down our upstairs hallway until my brain felt tired. The next day I often would sleep through high school classes I found boring but somehow still managed to get As. I was told that I wrote great papers in AP English, but I had no organization. To which I replied in my head, "But that's how my brain works."

It was during my freshman year of college at the University of South Carolina when I really started to struggle with everything. No matter how hard I tried, I couldn't keep up with schoolwork or sorority chapter meetings, and there was no way I could keep my dorm room any level of clean. I started to suspect I had ADHD because my freshmen year roommate had it and we were two peas in a pod. So I brought it up with my eating disorder therapist who started the evaluation process with me.

As for my complicated relationship with food, that started my junior year of high school. It was a way to deal with the chaos in my mind and to reclaim "control" when my family moved from Georgia to North Carolina. I became hyperfixated on being as "healthy" (read: thin) as possible. This was my gateway to developing anorexia.

Over the next eight years, my eating disorder shifted to binge eating and then bulimia. I found myself trapped in what I now realize was the ADHD binge/restrict cycle of not eating enough during the day and bingeing at night, as well as overexercising to "make up" for my binge eating.

Over those years, my ADHD diagnosis, therapy, and medication were very helpful in my healing journey. Getting my ADHD managed freed up the mental space I needed to work on healing my relationship with food and my body, but it wasn't until I discovered Intuitive Eating that I started to really understand the ways that ADHD impacted my relationship with food. Once I understood this, I was able to heal and find ease in my relationship with food, something I truly never imagined was possible.

Now I use my education, training as a dietician, and lived experienced as an ADHDer who was able to transform her relationship with food to show other ADHDers that healing is possible. If I was able to find the path that helped me heal what I thought would be a lifelong broken relationship, then I am confident that **you too can heal your relationship with food.**

What to Expect from This Book

This book is neurodiversity-affirming. You will gain a deeper understanding of how ADHD impacts your eating behaviors and learn to shed neurotypical expectations about feeding yourself. You'll discover practical tools and strategies to help you confidently eat in a way that works best for you and your brain.

This book takes a non-diet approach. This means you can expect to get encouragement and learn strategies to help you move away from restricting or avoiding foods and toward thinking about how you can give your body the nourishment it needs. We'll talk about the connection between eating disorders and ADHD and why it is so important to move away from restrictive dieting. We'll explore how to build better connections to your hunger and fullness cues and how to create an eating structure that works for you even if your body cues are unreliable. We'll discuss emotional regulation, eating for stimulation, and how to adopt a more flexible mindset around nourishing your body so you can finally move away from the all-or-nothing thinking that can feed the binge/restrict cycle.

In the final section, I'll share practical tools and strategies for working with your ADHD brain to make cooking and eating easier, from deciding what to eat to getting food on a plate to keeping up with the endless cycle of dishes. We will discuss how you can make accommodations to address executive function challenges in the kitchen so you can create a simple and practical framework to feed yourself that works for you and your unique needs. In the last chapter, I'll share simple, ADHD-friendly recipes for meals and snacks so you can start cooking.

What This Book Isn't

If you're looking for a book that makes the false promise that if you just eat a certain way your ADHD will be "healed," "cured," or "fixed," this is not that book. There are plenty of those types of books already. You can eat "clean," only buy organic, cut out sugar, gluten, and dairy, and take supplements, and you will still have ADHD.

Aside from making false promises, much of the advice in these books doesn't account for the fact that it takes a lot of time, money, and executive function to be able to cut out processed foods and make everything from scratch. As an ADHDer, I find it pretty ableist to push nutrition as a "cure" for something that doesn't have a cure and doesn't need to be cured, especially when it's written by an individual who doesn't live with ADHD.

How to Use This Book

As you read this book, there are few things I want you to keep in mind:

Adopt For-the-Most-Part Thinking

Throughout this book you will see recommendations like "eat every three or four hours." I want you to view these recommendations as *"for the most part*, eat every three or four hours." Why? Because you have ADHD, which means **you are consistently inconsistent** according to psychiatrist and ADHD expert Dr. Edward (Ned) Hallowell.

Prefacing your goals and behaviors with *for the most part* can help you break free of perfectionism and an all-or-nothing mindset. This adds flexibility and it will help you acknowledge that sometimes life can and will get in the way, but that doesn't mean you should stop trying to incorporate new, positive behaviors into your life.

Embrace Curiosity to Discover Your Why

This was one of the biggest mindset shifts that helped me heal my relationship with food. I used to believe that I needed to judge and berate myself for my eating mistakes. I thought that if I wasn't hard on myself that I'd slip. But as I explored Intuitive Eating, I learned to **approach my thoughts, feelings, and eating behaviors with curiosity instead of judgment.** Thinking this way will help you create space to figure out the "why" behind your eating behaviors and how you could do things differently in the future.

Let Go of Failure

Nourishing your body is not something you'll be graded on. View all of your eating experiences—past, present, and future—as opportunities to learn more about your body, the messages it gives you, and what works best for you. There is no one right way to nourish your body, so it's okay to experiment to figure these things out.

Remember, doing the same things over and over will lead to the same result and prevent you from shifting to a better way of eating and living. Think of your body as your home, one that will always be undergoing renovation.

There may be times when a strategy or tool works and other times when that same approach stops working. This is not a failure. It just means it's time to adjust. In fact, you'll probably need to swap out different tools and strategies regularly, because ADHD brains like novelty.

Give Yourself Grace and Try to Have Some Patience

For some, eating might be a lifelong struggle. Regardless of how long your relationship with food has been complicated, I invite you to give yourself grace for doing the best you can with the tools and resources you've had. Most nutrition advice does not accommodate ADHD-related challenges, so it makes sense that so many of us struggle with disordered eating and eating disorders.

It took me years to figure out my relationship with food. There were times when I thought it would be the monkey on my back my entire life. But I didn't give up and eventually reached the light at the end of the tunnel. I know that patience is not always a strength that we have as ADHDers, but I promise that, in this case, the end goal is worth the time and work.

It is my hope that reading this book will make life with ADHD a little easier and more fulfilling. I want you to feel confident that you are nourishing your body and brain in a way that works for you so you can feel your best—mentally and physically.

Ready to learn how to eat well with ADHD? Let's get started!

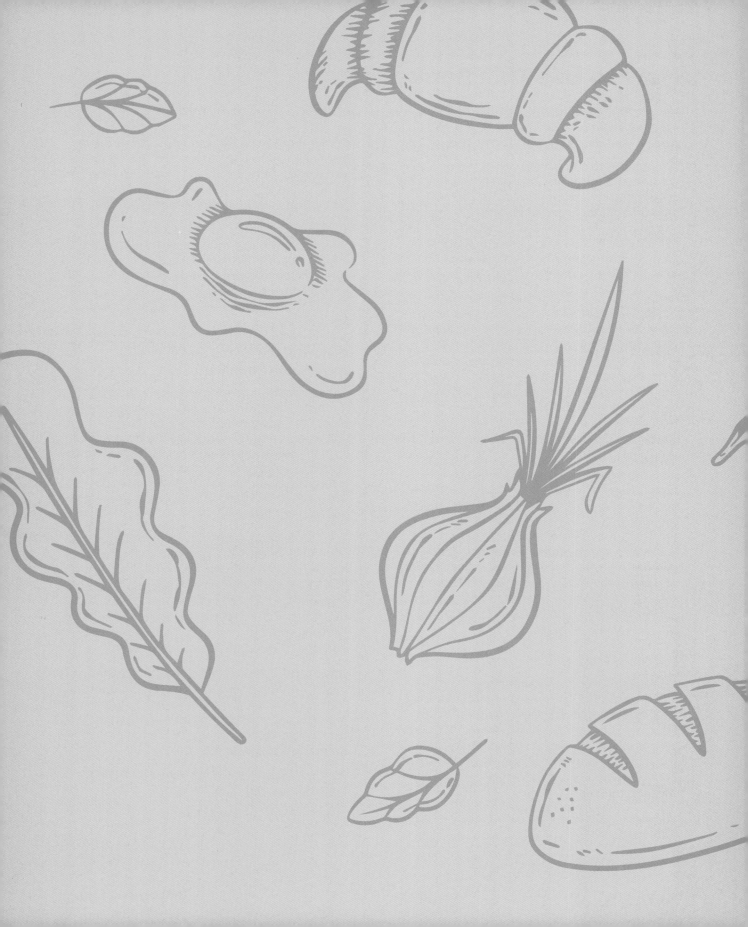

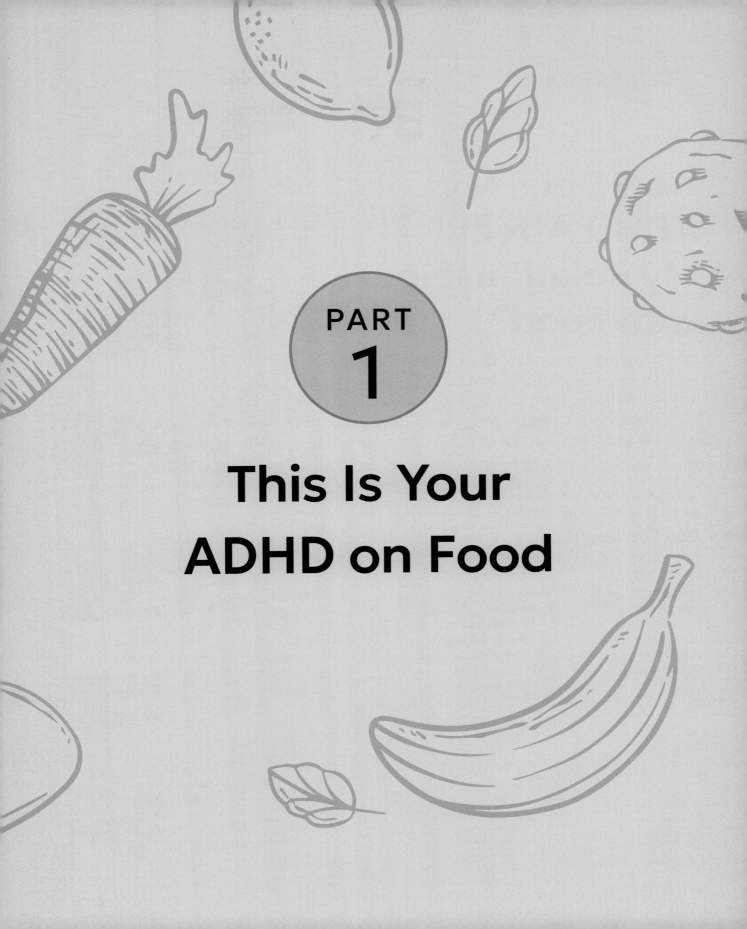

PART 1

This Is Your ADHD on Food

CHAPTER 1

How Does My ADHD Affect My Relationship with Food?

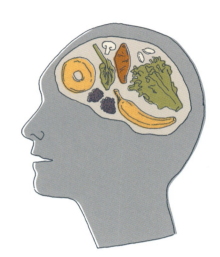

ADHD impacts every part of an ADHDer's life, including your relationship with food. Exploring how ADHD shows up in your life, especially if you were diagnosed at a later age, is like peeling an onion. As you peel back the layers of your life, you start to see all the different ways ADHD impacted you.

When I was diagnosed at 19, I understood that ADHD impacted my ability to pay attention, keep my apartment clean, and sit still for long periods of time. It wasn't until I got to graduate school that I realized how much ADHD impacted my ability to regulate my emotions and my relationships—including my super complicated relationship with food.

ADHDers struggle with following more healthful eating patterns because consistency is not our jam. For example, we know we need to eat fruits and veggies but not how to work with our brains to remember to eat them regularly or before they go bad in our fridges.

That's because many of the main "features" of ADHD—executive function differences, interoception challenges, the need for stimulation, taking medication, and emotional dysregulation—affect how you approach and interact with food. The medication(s) used to manage ADHD can also impact eating. We'll dive a lot deeper into these topics in future chapters, but here's a brief explanation for how these features show up when it comes to food.

Why Having ADHD Makes It Harder to Eat Well

Executive Function

Differences in executive function (EF), or the cognitive skills that help you plan, focus, problem solve, and achieve your goals, are at the heart of ADHD. These differences make it challenging to start, work on, and finish tasks.

When it comes to cooking and eating, we use executive function to decide what to eat, to plan meals, grocery shop, prepare food, cook, be aware of time, do the dishes, and keep our kitchen space semi-functional.

Dr. Thomas E. Brown, an expert on executive function and ADHD, breaks EF down into six different "buckets": activation, focus, effort, emotional regulation, memory, and action. In a person who does not have ADHD, these buckets usually work together quickly and unconsciously to help you with tasks such as grocery shopping and cooking. This is not the case with someone who has ADHD. The table on page 14 shows how ADHD can impact your relationship with food in each of these buckets.

No wonder ADHDers can find feeding themselves overwhelming! The good news? Throughout this book, we will discuss tools and strategies that can help manage these various executive function challenges.

Interoception Differences

If you struggle with recognizing when you're hungry, thirsty, full, or even when you need to pee, this is related to interoception differences. Interoception is being able to understand what is happening in our body, which is an important part of self-regulation. Interoception includes both the physical and emotional state of our bodies.

It can be challenging to give your body what it needs when you miss or confuse body cues and emotional states. This is one reason why ADHDers who don't take meds may find that they have no idea what it feels like to be hungry unless they're ravenous. In chapter 4, we will explore why it's so hard to listen to your body, what it feels like to be hungry or full, and strategies to improve interoceptive awareness.

The Quest for Dopamine

Dopamine and serotonin are naturally occurring chemicals that produce feelings of pleasure and calmness, respectively, in the human brain. ADHDers typically have low levels of dopamine. This means they are constantly looking for ways to increase their brain's dopamine levels or get stimulation. Food, especially simple carbs like sugar and baked goods, are quick and easy sources of dopamine. Eating these types of foods raises a person's dopamine as well as serotonin levels, making them feel calm and enjoyment, a welcome state of mind for anyone with ADHD.

But the inability to self-regulate (impulsivity), strong urge to combat boredom, and the desire for an immediate reward can lead to overeating. This is why ADHDers are more likely to struggle with overeating and binge eating. In Chapter 6, we will discuss in depth the ADHDer's quest for dopamine and how you can build a dopamine toolkit so that food is not your only source of stimulation.

Bucket	Function	The Affects of ADHD in Relation to Food
Activation	Organizing, prioritizing, and beginning the work	• You get stuck in freeze mode because you don't know where to begin with cooking. • A suggested cook time for a recipe is 30 minutes, but for you it takes an hour. • You delay eating until it's urgent and your body screams "I need food NOW!"
Focus	Giving and sustaining attention on a task	• You go into the kitchen to get a snack, but you get sidetracked by a package on the counter. • You regularly burn food because you forget about it or get distracted. • You get hyperfocused on your special interest and forget to eat or drink for 6+ hours.
Effort	Regulating alertness, sustaining effort, and processing speed	• You spend time making a meal plan, but don't follow it. • Keeping a food log feels like too much when you already struggle with simply remembering to eat and make food. • You can't shut off your mind at night so you stay up late watching TV and snacking.
Emotions	Manage frustration and modulate emotions	• You turn to food when feeling angry, depressed, stressed, lonely, etc. • You may also turn to food because you are afraid or don't know how to feel your feelings without them overcoming you. • Your short fuse leads to explosive responses when someone interrupts your cooking.
Memory	Utilize working memory and accessing recall	• You forget items at the grocery store or buy items you already have. • You need to reread recipe steps over and over. • You go all day without eating or drinking because you simply forgot.
Action	Monitor and self-regulate action	• You start cooking without first reviewing the directions or prepping everything you need. • You try to get through cooking as fast as possible and end up forgetting important steps in the process. • You find it difficult to cook regularly if you don't find it fun or enjoyable.

ADHD Medication

Stimulant medications are considered the gold standard for ADHD management, though there are also nonstimulant medications that can help. Both can affect appetite, but stimulants tend to have a bigger impact. Often, the decreased appetite from these medications leads to not eating enough or having inconsistent eating patterns during the day, followed by feeling ravenous and often bingeing or engaging in compensatory eating to make up for all the nutrition missed during the day. I call this the ADHD binge/restrict cycle, which you can experience whether you are medicated or unmedicated. This is one of the most common eating patterns I see with ADHDers.

Stimulants can be an incredible tool to help ADHDers stop self-medicating their ADHD with food. But medications can also make it easier to fall into the ADHD binge/restrict cycle because lack of appetite is one of the potential side effects. Throughout this book we will discuss medication and how to prevent or break free from the ADHD binge/restrict cycle.

Emotional Regulation

While emotional regulation challenges are not in the DSM-5, the diagnostic manual used to diagnose mental health conditions, most ADHD experts acknowledge it is a cornerstone of ADHD. This makes sense when you view ADHD through the lens of self-regulation, because the ability to regulate emotions is a key executive function. Eating can be a tool to help regulate emotions, but it can become problematic if it is your *only* tool to cope with your emotions.

Eating for emotional reasons and in the absence of hunger can also lead to overeating and binge eating. In Chapter 5, we will explore how food plays a role in emotional regulation, what to do if emotional eating is negatively impacting your relationship with food, and how to build an emotional coping toolkit.

Common Ways of Eating with ADHD: Which Is Your Avatar?

After working with hundreds of clients, I've identified common ways that ADHDers struggle when it comes to their relationship with food. The first five avatars represent each of these themes. You may relate to only one, a few, or all of these avatars. I've highlighted which chapters will be most helpful for each avatar. The final avatar, the Intuitive Eater, reflects the ideal relationship with food, which can be achievable after reading this book.

The Grazer

Grazers are ADHDers who feel as if they are constantly snacking or eating. The Grazer is usually either unmedicated or was diagnosed later in life. Grazers might be super frustrated that they are always boredom eating, mindlessly eating, or constantly eating even though they don't really feel hungry.

What Grazers may not realize is that they are eating this way as a form of self-medication. Food is giving their brain the dopamine it needs. Grazers may not know how real physical hunger feels because hunger is not the driving force in their eating. That driving force is the quest for dopamine. Grazers never really let themselves get hungry and they don't really know what fullness feels like except when they're stuffed. Grazers stop when the food is gone not when they feel full.

The Grazer tends to not have much of a plan around what or when they are eating, so they rely on a lot of snacks, delivery, and fast foods. They also like carbs, especially sweets and salty/crunchy foods, because they make their ADHD brain happy. If Grazers start meds, they may find that the grazing instinct disappears . . . at least while they are on medication. If you are a Grazer, you will benefit from chapters 3, 6, and 9.

The Binge/Restrictor

The Binge/Restrictor may feel as if they are either eating nothing or eating everything. There's a whole list of reasons they might find themselves in this eating pattern. It may show up as not eating much or at all during the day and bingeing or engaging in compensatory eating at night. This may be because medications suppress the appetite, they forget to eat, don't have enough time to eat, lose track of time/hyperfocus, or are trying to "make up" for eating "too much" the night before. Binge/Restrictors really want to be able to end the day

without binge eating. If you are stuck in this cycle, you will most likely benefit from chapters 3, 4, 5, and 6.

The Perfectionist

The Perfectionist's hyperfixation is eating healthy, dieting, and trying to be as healthy as possible. These ADHDers consider themselves professional trackers of what they eat. This may even become a disordered eating behavior.

Perfectionists like using a tracking system, whether it's calories or macros, because they don't trust themselves to know what, when, or how to eat. They get so much praise from others about their "perfect" eating that this might even become part of their identity.

But while these ADHDers come across as perfectionists with their eating, behind closed doors they are out of control around food. Perfectionists might secretly grab fast food on their way home from work and make an extra stop to throw out the "evidence" so no one will know. Or they might tell friends they have a migraine so they can't hang out, when in reality they're home, binge eating pizza, ice cream, and potato chips in front of the TV.

This may leave Perfectionists feeling frustrated, ashamed, and unsure what to do to fix it, because they can't let go of trying to be perfect, even though there is no one "perfect" way to eat. They may put so many spoons toward diet and exercise that they don't have a lot of spoons left. Perfectionists want to be able to access the energy they put into perfect eating for other areas of their lives. If this sounds like you, see chapters 2, 4, 5 and 8.

Takeout Queen or King

For Takeout Queens or Kings, the process of cooking isn't exciting, they don't have the time or cooking skills, or they just get so overwhelmed in the kitchen that they opt for spending three times the money on delivery and fast food. These ADHDers also may struggle with time management and use most of their spoons at work, so by the time they get home, they're too tired to cook.

Unfortunately, eating takeout constantly comes with a big ADHD tax and a heaping helping of shame, because they think they "should" be able to find the time, energy, and executive function to cook. Takeout Queens or Kings might be intimidated by the grocery store or kitchen because they never really learned how to navigate these spaces. Or they don't find cooking rewarding, so their brain screams NO THANK YOU at the thought of regularly cooking for themselves.

Another problem? Their taste buds have gotten so adjusted to eating highly palatable, delicious food from restaurants and fast food that when they try to cook, it always seems to fall short. Chapters 4 and 8 will likely be helpful for Takeout Queens and Kings.

The Selective Eater

Selective Eaters may have a lot of sensory sensitivities with food, hate being called "picky" eaters, or feel embarrassed because people tell them they "have the palette of a five-year-old." They've probably had to deal with a ton of comments around why they won't eat or even just take one bite. Often, Selective Eaters prefer beige and/or processed foods such as chicken nuggets, mac n' cheese, or whatever they ate as kids because these foods are safe and predictable in terms of taste and texture. Fruits and veggies are the Selective Eaters' enemy, even though they know they'd probably feel better if they ate more of them. Their tastebuds just don't like it.

Selective Eaters may be uninterested in food and feel shame for not enjoying food the way other people do. They might not eat out because of their limited palate or preferences. It's possible that their sensory aversions to food and potential food-related trauma may even lead them to develop an eating disorder called avoidant/restrictive food intake disorder (ARFID). See the next section to learn more about eating disorders. Chapter 7 will be helpful if you resonate with this avatar.

The Intuitive Eater

My hope is that this book will help you transform your relationship with food so you can become an Intuitive Eater! Intuitive Eaters have rebuilt trust that their bodies can tell them what, when, and how much to eat, or they have external supports that help with these things. These external supports or accommodations are not a way to "control" eating; rather, they are intended to support them with eating enough and eating regularly.

As a result, Intuitive Eaters feel at ease around all foods. They don't deprive themselves of foods they enjoy. They consider what they can ADD to their plates to promote satisfaction and add nutrition. Intuitive Eaters don't get stuck in the binge/restrict cycle. They can finally keep their "binge" foods in the house without fear they'll overindulge on them. These ADHDers match their energy or executive function with what they're cooking. Intuitive Eaters no longer feel pressure to eat "perfectly" or to fad diet. You'll learn more about this in the next chapter.

Except for the Intuitive Eater, in one way or another all of these avatars have an unmanageable relationship with food and eating well. But sometimes, this can become more serious and morph into an eating disorder.

ADHD and Eating Disorders

Eating disorders (ED) are incredibly complex and do not have a singular cause. ADHD is one factor that can increase the risk of developing an eating disorder. Another factor is engaging in dieting to lose weight. In fact, this is actually the strongest predictor of whether or not someone will develop an eating disorder.

Behind opioid overdoses, eating disorders are the second most deadly mental health condition. Yet, society has normalized engaging in behaviors that massively increase the odds of developing an ED. Some of these behaviors include avoiding certain foods or food groups, intentionally skipping meals, and engaging in compensatory behaviors to "make up" for what you've eaten. It's so pervasive that one study found **upward of 75 percent of women between the ages of 25 and 45 reported disordered eating or symptoms consistent with an eating disorder.**

ADHDers are at a significantly higher risk of developing an eating disorder compared to folks without ADHD. This is likely due to the need for stimulation, the hallmarks

How Diet Culture Impacts ADHDers's Relationships with Food

Diet culture is a system of beliefs that values thinness, appearance, and body shape. It oppresses folks, often from marginalized communities, who do not match this version of "health." But thinness does not equate to health. Not every thin person is healthy and not every person in a larger body is unhealthy. Diet culture has normalized recommending disordered eating behaviors to folks in larger bodies for the sake of shrinking their body. Body diversity exists and is a beautiful thing. We are all not meant to have the same hair, eyes, or height. So why would our body size and shape be any different?

Unfortunately, ADHDers are not immune to diet culture and are in fact more likely to engage in fad or crash diets than neurotypical people. The novelty of fad diets and their promises of quick (but unsustainable) results make them more appealing to ADHD brains that like immediate rewards.

Diet and wellness culture is *everywhere*—it permeates TV shows, movies, social media, magazines, and even our health guidelines. In 2023, the weight loss industry reached a new high of $89.9 billion in the United States alone. Yet, research shows that 80 percent of dieters regain lost weight within five years, and weight cycling, or losing and regaining weight, is associated with a higher risk of death. **Diets just don't work.**

Being truly healthy is more complicated than just following a diet as a means to control your body size. It means creating new lifelong habits, including eating nutritious foods, managing stress, getting enough sleep, moving your body in ways you enjoy, taking medications (if needed), moderating alcohol consumption, and kicking bad habits like smoking. It also means acknowledging the social determinants of health and how those factors may help or prevent you from being able to do these things.

of ADHD—hyperactivity, impulsivity, and inattention—along with self-loathing, distress, and the feeling of being unable to control eating behaviors. All of these traits mean ADHDers have the perfect storm for developing an ED. **Studies show the risk of developing an ED is three to five times higher for ADHDers.**

Developing an eating disorder absolutely sucks. While recovery is 100 percent possible, you never completely get rid of that voice in your head. If you overeat or even binge one night, then that voice might say, "You should skip breakfast." Or the voice might pop up during a particularly stressful time in life to try to convince you to go back to harmful behaviors to regain "control" in your life. But you can learn to put distance between you and those thoughts and learn strategies to disengage from your ED triggers.

As someone in recovery, I don't want other ADHDers (or really anyone) to experience the anguish, suffering, and despair that comes with an ED. Managing ADHD and usually at least one other mental health condition, such as depression or anxiety, is challenging enough. This is why I am so passionate about not dieting with the goal of weight loss. You can focus on your health and live healthfully without having to diet.

You can learn to make good choices for yourself not because you "should" but because it's what aligns with your values and makes you feel good. But this can be difficult with all the media noise about losing weight.

What's the Difference between Disordered Eating and an Eating Disorder?

Disordered eating is usually defined as irregular eating patterns that do not quite fit the criteria for an eating disorder diagnosis. These patterns tend to be less frequent and less severe than an ED. Often, people engaging in disordered eating behaviors are doing so to lose weight or for "health." These behaviors tend to be restrictive, compulsive, irregular, and inflexible.

But for ADHDers, disordered eating can be an unintentional consequence of ADHD. Disordered eating behaviors can include skipping meals, avoiding certain foods or food groups, inflexibility around what or when you'll eat, frequent dieting, binge eating, and using medications or supplements for the purpose of controlling weight.

Signs and symptoms of disordered eating include:

- Yo-yo dieting and weight fluctuations
- Feelings of guilt or shame when unable to maintain strict rules
- Feeling a loss of control around food
- Engaging in behaviors to "make up" for eating "bad" food
- Food noise, or a preoccupation with food, weight, and body image that negatively impacts quality of life
- Only eating "clean" or healthy foods
- Binge eating

When disordered eating behaviors become more severe, persistently interfere with eating patterns, and cause significant distress, they can become an eating disorder. Like ADHD, eating disorders also have genetic predispositions. Eating disorders include binge eating disorder, bulimia nervosa, anorexia nervosa, and avoidant/restrictive food intake disorder (ARFID).

Binge eating and bulimia are the two eating disorders most strongly associated with ADHD. ARFID is often discussed as an ED that kids and people with autism experience, but as awareness about AFRID grows, it has been linked to adults and ADHDers. Researchers and providers are realizing that those who are neurodivergent don't just grow out of "picky eating," and this can lead to lifelong challenges with eating that have nothing to do with body size or appearance. For more information on ARFID, see the sidebar on page 88.

If you struggle with disordered eating or an eating disorder, please seek out support from your health practitioner, a dietitian, therapist, or psychologist. Professionals who are neurodiversity-affirming, anti-diet, or embrace the Health at Every Size® (HAES®) philosophy can provide the support you need to help you improve your relationship with food and your body.

Intersections of Ableism and Anti-Fat Bias

The negative messages around fatness and neurodivergence are very similar. Both ADHDers and folks in larger bodies are viewed as "lazy," or "careless," with a "need to be fixed or cured." ADHD and body fat are often viewed as separate from a person instead of part of their identity. ADHDers who live in a larger body are more likely to seek out the thin ideal to counter negative assumptions about their ADHD.

This book may force you to challenge internalized ableism and anti-fat bias. If you aren't able to accept that your brain works differently and that you will need different tools and support from your non-ADHD peers, it's likely that you may continue to struggle with food and other areas of your life. The same is true if you aren't able to accept that all bodies—including your own—deserve dignity and respect.

What Does a Healthy Relationship with Food Look Like?

When a potential client shares, "I want a healthy relationship with food," my follow-up is, "What does a healthy relationship with food look like for you?" Sometimes they know because they've been thinking about it or exploring recovery. But more often, a slightly confused look comes over their face and they respond, "Well, I don't really know." If this is you, it's okay! Hopefully by the end of this book, you will be able to confidently define what a healthy relationship with food means for you.

Bottom line? **A healthy relationship with food is one that is free of guilt and shame around what, when, why, and how you eat.**

It's working with your ADHD brain to come up with a plan so that eating doesn't feel like a full-time job. It is choosing to not engage in restrictive eating behaviors as punishment. It is acknowledging that diets do not work and choosing not to do them. It is having rules or boundaries with food that stem from a place of love instead of a place of fear. It is using your knowledge about nutrition and your inner wisdom about what food feels good in your body to guide your food choices.

If your only goal with food is to shrink your body, then you aren't really teaching yourself how to live a healthful life.

What Would You Like Your Relationship with Food to Look Like?

Before we move on, I invite you to do some reflecting on your own relationship with food. I encourage you to write your answers down so that you can consider them more carefully:

Which avatar(s) do you resonate with? What are your biggest challenges related to food? Do they stem from a history of dieting or disordered eating or only from ADHD? How would your eating be different if you were able to let go of dieting and embrace working with your ADHD brain to remove the chaos and feelings of being overwhelmed and shamed from your relationship with food?

Most importantly, what you would like your relationship with food to look like?

CHAPTER 2

Intuitive Eating for ADHD

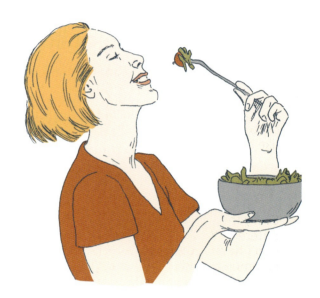

Somewhere toward the end of my undergrad years and the beginning of grad school, I first encountered Intuitive Eating (IE). I found it thanks to dietitians on Instagram and remember feeling both curious and extremely resistant to it.

These dietitians talked about eating what you want, when you want, and that you can listen and trust your body about what, when, and how much to eat. Honestly, I thought it was a bunch of woo-woo BS. I thought that's great for them, but I could *never* trust or listen to my body.

That's because when I take ADHD medication, it disrupts my hunger cues and makes knowing what to eat and when very confusing. I also felt that if I tried IE while on my meds, it somehow meant that I was cheating the whole process. I share this because I know so many ADHDers feel this way when they initially learn about IE.

Intuitive eating is the polar opposite of everything we've ever been told when it comes to food and our bodies. Diet culture teaches us that our bodies cannot be trusted and that we need to rely on things like calorie counting or tracking macros instead of listening to our bodies.

Why IE Works for ADHDers

Diets are rigid, require you to remember a lot of rules every time you make a food choice, and often require you to track what you're eating, which can make eating feel even more overwhelming. Diets require a level of consistency that is not realistic for most ADHDers. This often leads to feeling like a failure, when in reality it's the unsustainable diet that has failed you.

In contrast, Intuitive Eating prioritizes flexibility. It encourages you to adapt the 10 principles (see page 25) to fit your unique lifestyle, cooking skills, and needs. It considers both your emotional and physical health. It encourages you to let go of restrictive food rules, shame, and guilt. It teaches you how to build a better connection to the messages your body is giving you and to use that information to guide your food choices.

I don't know about you, but eating nutritious foods makes me feel good. Usually when folks feel "good" on a diet it's because they are eating more nutrient-dense foods. It's a lot easier to eat nutritious foods when your motivation is because it feels good and not because you "should." Shoulding yourself never leads to sustainable, long-term behavior changes.

IE acknowledges that you are the expert on your body because you are really the only person who knows what hunger/fullness feels like in your body and how certain foods make you feel. I find IE helps remove shame and guilt around eating, and you can't fail at it, which can improve your self-esteem.

IE also embraces the belief that all foods can fit into a healthful eating pattern, which I find helpful, as many ADHDers experience sensory sensitivities, difficulties eating on meds, and find cooking overwhelming.

Your IE Journey

Everyone's timeline on an IE journey will be different. While this is an inward journey, you don't have to do it on your own. In fact, I find community and professional support is helpful not only for improving your relationship with food but also with managing your ADHD.

I went solo during the two years of my grad program and nine months of my dietetic internship. Looking back, I really wish I'd reached out to a dietitian or therapist who could have helped me work through this process.

But I didn't think I'd find support. I was wrong. It doesn't matter what you do for a living, how old you are, or how long you've struggled with food; it's never too late to get support for your eating (and ADHD).

In this chapter, we are going to explore why traditional diets don't work for ADHDers (or anyone, really), what Intuitive Eating is, what it is not, the risks, the benefits, how to adapt this framework to your brain, and resources if you want to learn more.

Society is Diet-Crazy and Fatphobic

Society tells people at a young age, especially women, to shrink our bodies at all costs. To try to fit into the mold that society tells us is attractive, to emulate airbrushed models and try to become perfect. Often this comes at the expense of our mental health, physical health, and happiness.

As Christy Harrison, registered dietitian and author of *Anti-Diet* and *The Wellness Trap* explains, dieting is a way to keep you "distracted from your pleasure, your purpose, and your power." While I do not know what it is like to live in a larger body, I can promise you that no matter how small I've gotten, it was never small enough.

If you live in a larger body, you probably experience weight stigma from partners, friends, family, coworkers, and even medical providers. If you've lost weight, you may have been treated differently or maybe navigated the world more easily. But if you have to engage in disordered behaviors like restrictive dieting to maintain that weight, it may not be the ideal weight for you. You can't fight your genetics, and you can't white-knuckle your way through life to maintain a weight you weren't meant to be.

What Exactly Is Intuitive Eating (IE)?

Intuitive Eating is a non-diet approach to nutrition that it is weight-neutral. It's a lifelong way of eating that finds the middle ground between being overly restrictive and eating whatever you want, regardless of how it makes you feel. Intuitive Eating teaches you how to trust your body to guide you to make food choices that make you feel good, without judgment or the influence of diet culture. Instead of shaming you for "bad" food choices, IE helps you understand why you might turn to food when you are not hungry.

Intuitive Eating was created by two dietitians, Evelyn Tribole and Elyse Resch. It is a self-care-focused framework for eating that integrates instinct, emotion, and rational thought. It means being able to enjoy a cookie without guilt or having chips with guacamole and carrots for a snack because you know that chips by themselves don't fill you up unless you eat A LOT. It's also stopping when you're full instead of when your plate is clean.

It's honoring your cravings without guilt because you know that they will turn into uncontrollable cravings and possibly binge eating if you don't. It's realizing that when you actually tune into your body, it not only craves fun foods, such as ice cream or french fries, but also nutritious foods like a crunchy apple or refreshing salad. Intuitive Eating is not eating what you want, regardless of how it will make you feel or how it will impact your health.

I think of it as removing the "shoulds" around eating and exploring with curiosity what will make you feel your best mentally and physically. There is no one "right" way to eat intuitively. This approach creates space for you to adapt to meet your needs throughout life because this changes, often on a daily basis.

There are over 200 published peer-reviewed studies on IE. Benefits of Intuitive Eating include:

- reduced depression and anxiety
- improved body satisfaction
- greater self-acceptance
- improved quality of life
- decreased binge eating
- decreased restrained eating/dieting
- improvements to total cholesterol and LDL cholesterol
- lower blood pressure
- improved blood sugar regulation
- improved interoception
- more satisfaction with life
- decreased emotional eating

Unlike a traditional diet, you cannot fail at IE. Every eating experience is an opportunity for you to learn more about what your body is telling you and rebuild trust with your body.

The 10 Principles of Intuitive Eating

There are 10 guiding principles in the IE framework. These principles are not steps or commandments. They are a framework designed to help you become more flexible, intuitive, and at ease with your relationship with food and with your body. Although you may want to start by working with one principle, all of them work together to promote satisfaction and pleasure.

True Intuitive Eating leaves you feeling comfortably full and satisfied after eating without feelings of guilt or shame. These principles work in two ways. First, they help you build better connection to the physical sensations or messages your body sends, such as hunger or stress, so that you can meet your physical or psychological needs.

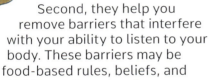

Second, they help you remove barriers that interfere with your ability to listen to your body. These barriers may be food-based rules, beliefs, and thoughts. For ADHDers, these barriers can also include executive function challenges, interoception differences, and ADHD medications.

Principle 1: Rejecting the Diet Mindset

IE is not a diet. A large body of research shows that diets do not work long-term. Most people aren't able to lose weight and keep it off. Instead they tend to gain back even more weight, which is beyond counterproductive.

If you have a history of disordered eating or an eating disorder, then it's important to know that dieting and restricting are not recommended. Binge eating is the most common response to physical and mental diet restrictions (as well as our need for stimulation, emotional reasons, and other factors). For me, the more I restricted and tried to control my eating, the worse my bingeing became. Chronic dieting and restriction can also make it more difficult to pick up on your body cues.

Traditional diets require a level of consistency that is not realistic for most ADHDers because we tend to approach everything with an all-or-nothing mindset. If you're anything like I was before I started IE, you're either dieting or eating whatever you want, no matter how you feel. When a diet is new or exciting, it's easy to stick to. But once the novelty wears off, you're back to your old behavior. Constantly going on and off diets or jumping from one fad diet to the next can lead to weight cycling or yo-yo weight. This has been found to be more dangerous to your health than simply remaining at a higher weight.

Letting go of the belief that you need to follow a bunch of food rules creates space for you to explore what works best for you to feel your best.

Principle 2: Honoring Your Hunger and Principle 5: Feeling Your Fullness

IE is sometimes oversimplified as "eat when you are hungry and stop when you are full." But honoring the signals your body sends you when you are hungry or full are only two of the ten principles. This oversimplification can make IE seem impossible for ADHDers who struggle to recognize body cues or take meds that that make it difficult to sense those body cues. Overall, the goal of honoring your hunger and feeling your fullness is to eat regularly and enough to prevent you from falling into the extreme ends of hunger and fullness.

When working with clients who are new to IE, I tell them to focus on eating every three to four hours instead of solely relying on hunger/fullness cues. It can also be helpful to create an external structure, like setting an alarm, to make it easier to check in with your body so you can learn what hunger feels like. This makes it easier to meet your needs before they become too uncomfortable to ignore. Chapter 3 will show you more ways to do this and begin practicing it in real life.

Principle 3: Make Peace with Food

In my personal experience and in the work I've done with clients, this is one of the more challenging principles. It means giving yourself unconditional permission to eat *with attunement*. This principle promotes food neutrality—or the belief there are no "good" or "bad" foods.

For ADHDers, this principle may involve making peace with your sensory preferences and eating behaviors. You are allowed to have food preferences. It's okay if you don't eat everything or if you only like a food when it is prepared in certain ways.

For example, I don't like and will not eat steamed veggies because they are too mushy. Instead, I enjoy roasted and raw veggies because they're nice and crunchy. You may have to accept that you can get hyperfixated on a food or that you need to use more convenience foods, like individual-size yogurt cups, to lower the barrier to eating.

Placing a moral value on food adds unnecessary shame and judgment about your food choices, which you're likely to internalize. So, when you eat a "bad" food, you tell yourself you are "bad," and that you deserve to feel "bad."

It's true that different foods like fruits and vegetables and complex carbs and protein provide more sustained energy and important nutrients. While these types of food are more nourishing for our bodies, other foods like your mom's homemade apple pie or the pizza you eat while catching up with your friends are more nourishing for our souls. Both are important.

The process of making peace with food is called habituation. It's having repeated exposures to foods to remove their sense of novelty. If you previously restricted a food, habituation shows your brain that these foods are no longer scarce.

I have my clients make a list of their forbidden or shame foods and rank them from least to greatest in terms of how distressing it would be to eat that food. Then, we work through the list, one food at a time, creating positive eating experiences to normalize the food before moving to the next one.

Usually, there is a mental shift when you realize these foods are no longer off limits. From this point you can trust your body to tell you when to stop eating so you don't have to work through every food on that list. This process can be complicated and challenging, so you may want to consider working with a registered dietitian or therapist.

Principle 4: Discovering the Satisfaction Factor

This principle focuses on how you can honor your sensory preferences with food and create a conducive eating environment. Together these two things make eating satisfying and enjoyable. I think of **the satisfaction factor as the mental component to fullness.**

If you don't allow yourself to eat foods you enjoy or find ways to make nutritious foods taste good, then you will keep eating around your cravings. One of my big aha moments came after I was craving chocolate chip cookies, but I told myself I "shouldn't." So instead, I binged on all the "healthier" options, hoping to satisfy my craving. But it didn't work. So, I made and ate most of the cookies and felt STUFFED. I realized afterward that if I had just eaten the cookies that I truly wanted, even if I ate all of them, I still would have eaten less food and felt less uncomfortably full.

When you eat your favorite foods, I want you to consider what sensory qualities contribute to an enjoyable eating experience. How do taste, texture, aroma, temperature, appearance, and your eating environment contribute to satisfaction? Also consider who you are eating it with. How can you incorporate these factors into other food moments to promote more satisfying eating experiences?

Principle 5: See Principle 2 for details.

Principle 6: Challenge the Food Police

The Food Police is your inner food critic. It is the sum of the messages you've heard from food companies, the media, friends, family, and even strangers about the "right" way to eat. This principle helps you identify cognitive distortions you have about your food rules. It also helps you unlearn harmful beliefs around food that you've learned from external sources. For neurodivergent folks, neurotypical eating standards can also be challenging, such as having to eat without distractions to eat mindfully or spending hours prepping a Sunday meal to eat healthfully. You can start to challenge the Food Police by identifying unhelpful rules and beliefs such as:

- I shouldn't eat pasta because it has too many carbs and will make me gain weight.
- No eating after 8:00 pm, even if I'm hungry.
- I need to skip breakfast to "make up" for binge eating at night.
- If I eat one "bad" food, then I might as well say screw it and eat whatever.

Explore your thoughts and behaviors with curiosity instead of judgment. When you let go of the judgment, you can create space to gain a greater understanding of the reasoning behind your eating. This can help you actually find solutions to make lasting change.

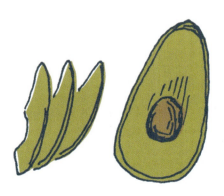

Principle 7: Cope with Your Emotions with Kindness

This principle is all about understanding the ways in which you may turn to or rely on food to cope with your emotions. It's acknowledging that eating may be a coping skill and that it is normal and okay to eat for emotional reasons. For some ADHDers, eating for stimulation or to regulate your emotions may be a form of self-care that ensures you eat when your physical hunger cues are unreliable. This is why I approach eating for stimulation the same way the authors of IE approach "emotional eating."

This means accepting that we may use food this way, but it's also important to find other coping strategies such as breathing exercises, venting to verbally process emotions, having a solo dance party in your living room, or tapping into your creative side to express your feelings through painting or drawing.

Before you can cope with your emotions, you have to learn how to feel your feelings. This means learning to tolerate intense, uncomfortable feelings instead of turning to food or restricting food as a way to cope. We will talk in chapter 5 all about using food to cope with your emotions, and in chapter 6 we will chat about using food for dopamine.

Principle 8: Respect Your Body

All bodies, regardless of shape or size, deserve dignity and respect. This includes your body. So many of us have spent years, decades, or even most of our lives hating our bodies. The goal of principle 8 is not to love your body but to learn how to care for and respect your lifelong home so you can live a fulfilling, meaningful life.

Accepting yourself instead of focusing on diets can also create space for other more fun and interesting activities. It's a lot easier to be present in the moment when you aren't stressed over your weight, keeping mental track of how much or how little you ate, or what you need to do to "make up" for what you ate.

The journey to accepting your neurodivergence can be a valuable tool to help with body acceptance and vice versa.

Tips for body acceptance:

- Diversify your social media feed by following accounts of people of all shapes and sizes.
- Unfollow or mute accounts that make you feel bad about yourself.
- Read books, listen to podcasts, or watch YouTube videos about body acceptance and anti-fat bias.
- Seek out health care providers who embrace Health at Every Size® (HAES®)
- Buy clothes that fit and showcase your incredible personality.
- Set boundaries with family, friends, partners, and coworkers around diet and body talk. If they don't respect your boundaries, don't give them as much or any of your time.

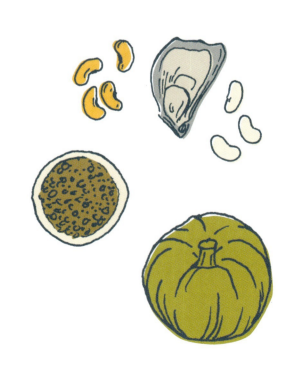

Principle 9: Movement— Feel the Difference

This principle focuses on how you can engage in regular movement that you enjoy to feel strong and energized. Throughout this book I will use movement instead of exercise because it is about exploring ways you can move your body more throughout the day, which may not include what we consider "exercise." I really believe it is important to find movement you enjoy that also honors your sensory needs, mobility, energy levels, and attention span.

Give yourself permission to engage in whatever movement feels accessible to you. Again, this doesn't have to be traditional "exercise" at a gym. There are so many short-term and long-term benefits to moving your body, including helping with managing ADHD. You do not have do an intense workout, move for a certain amount of time, do it at the gym, or sweat for it to "count." Maybe movement looks like joining a pickleball league with your friends, using a VR headset to gamify movement, taking an aerial circus class, or running around with your kids in the backyard.

Principle 10: Gentle Nutrition

This is the last principle in Intuitive Eating for a reason. We are so conditioned to diet that it can be very easy to turn Intuitive Eating into a set of rules if you jump to gentle nutrition before you've unlearned all of your dieting beliefs, focused on healing your relationship with food, and built body trust. Once you've done those things, then you can start focusing on how to add more nutrition into your eating or making more healthful choices without morphing it into another diet. You'll learn more about this principle in chapter 7.

Myths About Intuitive Eating, Debunked

Like any change, switching to Intuitive Eating can be challenging in the beginning. It can take time to become more attuned to your body needs. For ADHDers, who tend to be impatient and want immediate results, this can be frustrating.

While researching the so-called "cons" of IE, I kept seeing "You may not lose weight." But I cannot stress enough that this is *not* the purpose or intention of this eating framework. It's understandable to want to lose weight when we've been programmed to believe that being thin is the secret to health and happiness. But believe me, you are so much more than your body size, and good health is far more satisfying than the number on the scale.

If you're still not convinced, here are five myths about switching to Intuitive Eating, debunked.

IE Doesn't Care about Nutrition or Health

This is simply false. In this framework, Gentle Nutrition is the last principle. Saying it is okay to eat a cookie without guilt is not anti-health. Health is not just your body size or physical health. It's also your mental and emotional health. Constantly stressing about your food choices, engaging in negative self-talk about your food choices, and depriving yourself of enjoyable eating experiences is also not great for your mental health.

I Won't Stop Eating

If you are coming off a period of restriction or deprivation, especially a long period, then you probably will experience stronger hunger pangs than normal and eat more food as a result. Dieting is basically a self-imposed famine. Your body doesn't know the difference between choosing to deprive yourself of energy and nutrients and not having access to food. So it responds in the same way.

Our ancestors basically lived on a binge/restrict cycle. When they got access to food, they ate as much as they could to store energy for when they didn't have access to food. You cannot override that biology with willpower. You have to teach your body and brain that you are safe and you can trust yourself with food.

I Can't Eat Intuitively Because I Have [Insert Health Condition]

If you have certain medical conditions, like type 2 diabetes or PCOS, then you may have to modify your eating to support managing your condition, which is also called Medical Nutrition Therapy (MNT). But this doesn't mean that you can't eat intuitively.

For example, if you have type 2 diabetes, you might try to cut out carbs only to find yourself stuck in a binge/restrict cycle with carbs, which will not help with managing blood sugar levels. With IE, you can explore how to eat regularly to keep your blood sugar stable and to prevent getting overly hungry, which can lead to binge eating. You can also focus on making peace with carbs and learn how to pair them with protein and fat to support stable blood sugar.

Basically, IE can help people attain autonomy within MNT guidelines to figure out what works for them to feel their best for the long-term. This can lead to sustainable behavior change instead of swinging between trying to take better care of yourself for a while and then saying "Forget it!" If you have a health condition and want to start IE, you may want to seek guidance from an Intuitive Eating dietitian first.

Not Enough Structure

Some folks feel like IE doesn't have enough structure and feels too free. But again, this is a flexible framework so you can explore how to create a structure that feels supportive for you. Some examples of structure could be eating every three to four hours or determining a minimum amount of food to eat each day or for meals or snacks.

If you are curious about this framework, please work with a dietitian or therapist to learn how to incorporate it into your life. Reading and consuming content is a start, but getting support from trained professionals is the next step. A dietitian or therapist can help you customize this framework to you, your brain, your lifestyle, and your needs.

I'll Just Eat "Junk" Food All Day Long

Remember, you have unconditional permission to eat with attunement. The attunement piece is so important. It means that you consider how food will make you feel and factor that into your food choices. I do not know a single person who feels good when they only eat cookies, chips, pizza, fries, fast food, or sugary sodas.

What would happen if you ate like that every day for a week? Do you think at some point you would want something more nutrient-dense? In the beginning phase of IE, it is normal to eat more of these foods. We call it the honeymoon phase. Interestingly, research shows Intuitive Eaters actually eat a wider variety of foods, including more fruits and veggies compared to dieters.

Intuitive Eating can be a life-changing way to approach food and take care of your physical, mental, and emotional health. It's a framework that you can adapt to your unique needs and brain, allowing you to feel at ease around all foods. IE can help you develop a better connection to your body so that you can meet your physical and psychological needs.

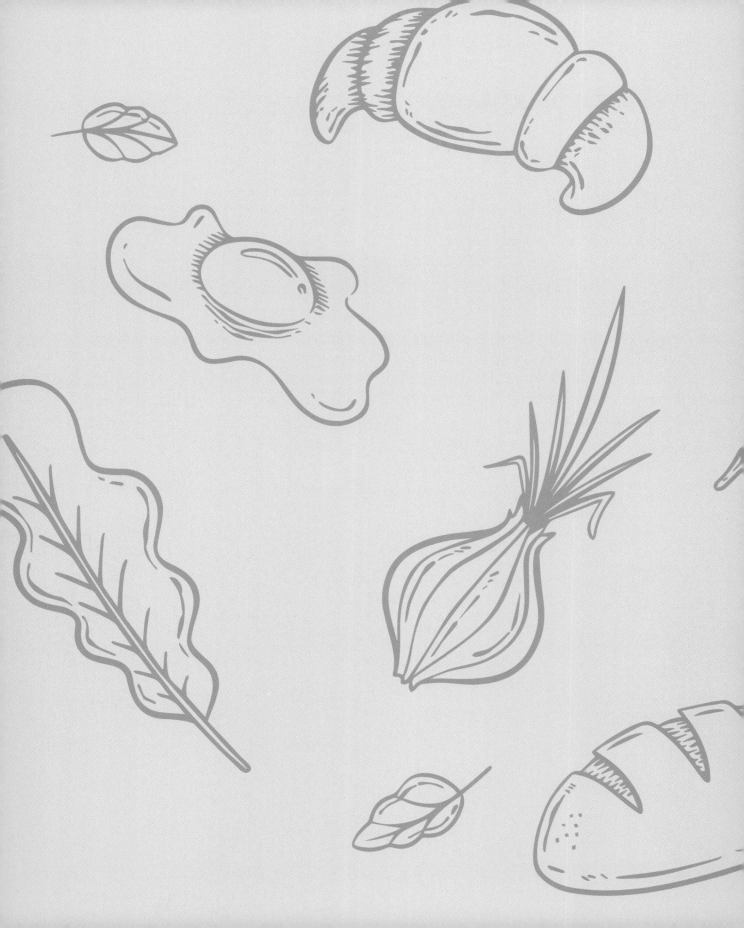

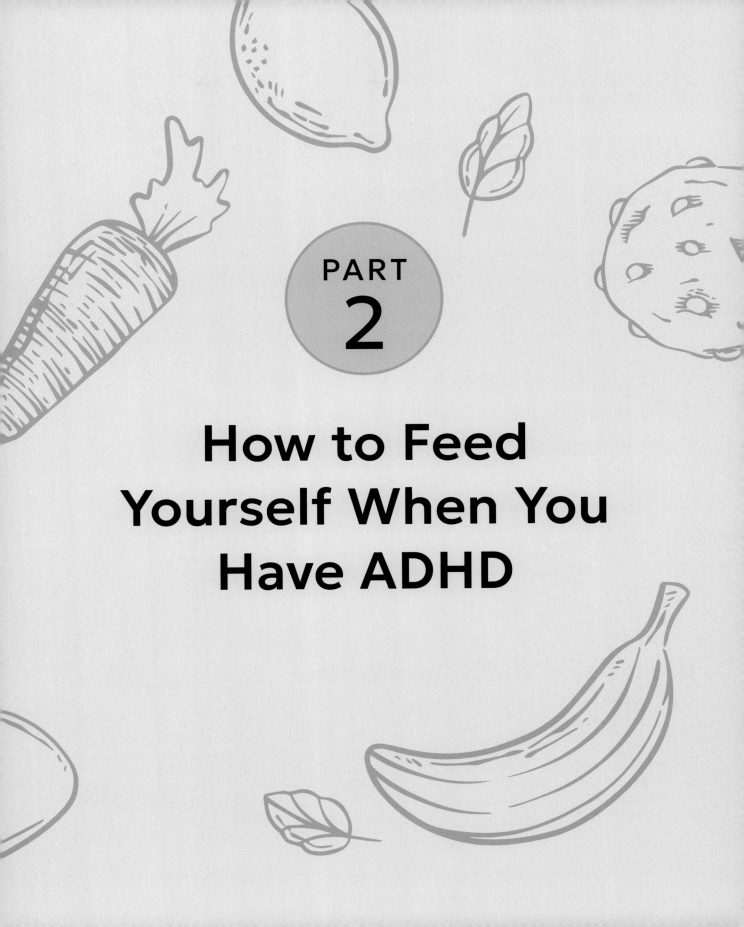

PART 2

How to Feed Yourself When You Have ADHD

CHAPTER 3

Why Is It So Hard for Me to Listen to My Body?

I can't tell you how many times ADHDers have told me "I don't really know how to tell when I'm hungry or full, except when I'm RAVENOUS or STUFFED." In this chapter we are going to discuss why it's so hard for ADHDers to listen to their bodies, how to tell when you're hungry and full, and what to do if you cannot. We'll also discuss ways to build a better connection with your body so you can listen to it and rebuild trust. But first, let's talk about what "listening to your body" even means.

What Is Interoceptive Awareness? How Does It Play a Role in Eating?

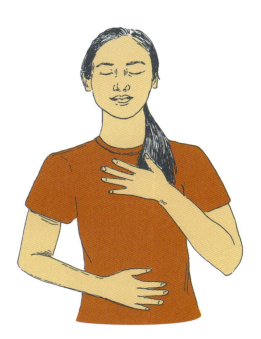

Interoception is often referred to as our eighth sense (taste, touch, sound, sight, hearing, vestibular, and proprioception are the other senses). It is defined as the perception of physical sensations related to internal organ function such as heartbeat, respiration, and satiety. Interoception also relates to the autonomic nervous system activity related to emotions. Basically, interoception is being able to understand what is happening in our body or our internal environment, which is important for self-regulation.

Recognizing Bodily Cues When You Have ADHD: Hunger

What comes to mind when you think about hunger? Where does it show up in your body? Most folks think of a growling stomach. But your stomach is not the only part of your body that can send you messages that you need food. In this section, we will explore different forms of hunger. In the book *Intuitive Eating*, authors Evelyn Tribole and Elyse Resch discuss five forms of hunger: biological, primal (also known as rebound), practical, emotional, and taste hunger. But I like to add another form of hunger: brain hunger.

All of these types of hunger are morally neutral and valid reasons to eat. I find that naming why you are hungry or the type of hunger you are experiencing can help prevent judging or beating yourself up for eating.

The better you become at identifying the different forms of hunger and eating more consistently, the easier it will be to determine why you want to eat. Contrary to popular diet culture advice, you don't have to be hungry enough to eat an apple to justify needing a snack.

Types of Hunger

You may have been told it's bad to eat for emotional reasons, for stimulation, or because your body is craving a specific food. But you're not a bad person for listening to your body. Demonizing other forms of hunger is not helpful because it adds shame and judgment to eating. There's nothing wrong with honoring these other forms of hunger if you know why you're choosing to eat and doing so with intention.

Physical or Biological Hunger

For ADHDers, I find that physical hunger cues are harder to recognize or might not even be something they experience. Biological hunger is another name for physical hunger. This form of hunger is what most people think of when their stomach growls. It's often the only form of hunger that is considered "acceptable."

You can experience physical hunger in different parts of your body. Some of the signs of physical hunger appear on page 37. (The italicized cues are hunger cues that exacerbate ADHD symptoms.)

As you can see, some of the signs of hunger can also be caused by other things. That's one reason why ADHDers can confuse these messages for something else. If you notice one of these physical hunger cues, then pause and prioritize eating something. Especially if it is an unpleasant hunger cue. If eating causes that cue to dissipate, then it's likely a hunger cue.

Hunger: On and Off Meds

ADHD meds, especially stimulants, can zap your appetite. But more often than not, when my clients start paying attention to their hunger cues, they experience a change in how they feel but don't connect it to being hungry. This is similar to confusing a headache as a sign that you need caffeine when you actually need food.

For this reason, it can be helpful to learn your hunger cues on and off meds. When my clients notice changes in mood or their ability to focus or concentrate suddenly gets more challenging, despite being medicated, more often than not eating helps get their mood, focus, or concentration back to baseline.

Remember that if you have days when you do not take your ADHD meds, it is normal to feel hungrier, especially if you are not eating enough on the days when you take your meds. You will also likely need to consider that your ADHD brain will want to seek out stimulation because your brain is not getting dopamine from your meds. When I do not take my meds, I find it helpful to remind myself to prioritize eating every three to four hours and work stimulating activities into my day to satisfy my ADHD brain.

Signs of Hunger for ADHD

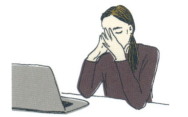

Lack of focus

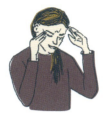

Headache

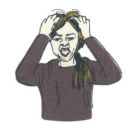

Irritability

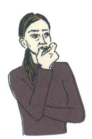

Anxiety

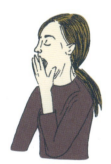

Fatigue

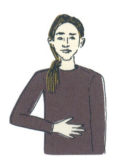

Growling stomach

Primal Hunger: The "Hunger Monster" or Rebound Hunger

This type of hunger can show up when you've gone too long without eating and suddenly feel *ravenous*. This insatiable and uncomfortable form of hunger tends to lead to a chaotic and urgent eating experience. This is a "Holy cow, I'm hungry and need food NOW" kind of hunger! In *Intuitive Eating*, this form of hunger is referred to as primal hunger.

Rebound hunger can happen as a result of intentional restriction such as dieting or struggling with an eating disorder. One example may be the weekly cycle of "doing good" all week and then bingeing on the weekends. You may have also experienced this type of hunger as part of food insecurity. This form of hunger is rooted in restriction—whether or not that restriction is intentional. When you are eating enough consistently, this type of hunger will likely not show up.

Rebound hunger is a survival mechanism for your body. Your body doesn't know the difference between self-imposed starvation (dieting), forgetting to eat all day, and being in a true famine. Rebound hunger is your body trying to make up for the nutrition and energy it didn't get all day or while you were restricting. So don't beat yourself up when the hunger monster shows up. Instead, try to practice gratitude that your body is taking care of you and explore what you can do differently in the future to keep the hunger monster away.

Practical Hunger

If you're an ADHDer who thinks you can't eat intuitively, then let's chat about how you can use practical hunger. Practical hunger is *key* for ADHDers who have unreliable hunger cues but still want to eat intuitively, because it allows you to pair your logic with your intuition. I've heard many ADHDers say, "If I just listened to my body, I would not eat all day and binge at night." Logically, you probably know this way of eating doesn't make you feel very great physically or mentally. So, instead of waiting until the hunger monster shows up to eat, you could choose to eat every few hours. Again, listening to your body is not just listening for physical hunger cues.

If you follow me on social media, I share about eating every three to four hours A LOT. Practical hunger can help you do this, despite having unreliable or unpredictable hunger cues. Establishing a more consistent eating pattern can help your body begin to anticipate when you will eat, which can help you reconnect with physical hunger cues. In chapter 4, we will discuss more of the benefits of eating more regularly. But I think it's helpful to view honoring practical hunger as an act of proactive self-care that keeps the hunger monster away.

Here's some examples of how to use practical hunger.

Emotional Hunger

Yes, it's normal and okay to eat for emotional reasons. Food factors into so many aspects of our lives. I'd argue that it's nearly impossible to separate emotions from food.

However, if food is your only tool to cope with your emotions, this can become problematic. If you're experiencing emotional hunger regularly, consider working with a therapist or counselor to develop other coping skills that will provide a safe way to process your emotions.

It can be easy to confuse emotional hunger for other forms of hunger, especially physical and rebound hunger. It can also trigger binge eating. But don't worry, we will talk more in-depth about emotional eating in chapter 5.

Brain Hunger

For ADHDers, I think eating for stimulation or dopamine needs its own hunger category. I

Physical Hunger Cues

Part of Body	Potential Hunger Cue
Head	**Pleasant:** start thinking about food, look forward to eating, increased salivation when thinking about food or when around food **Unpleasant:** ringing in ears, *cloudy thinking*, headache, *lack of concentration/focus/attention, inability to make decisions*, urgent and intense desire to eat, feeling ravenous, faint or lightheaded
Throat/esophagus	**Pleasant:** dull ache or gnawing sensation
Stomach	**Pleasant:** growling, rumbling, or gurgling sensation **Unpleasant:** gnawing, intense stomachache, emptiness
Body	**Unpleasant:** sweating, gas, digestive discomfort, overall lethargy
Mood	**Unpleasant:** *irritability/crankiness/hangry*, restlessness, discomfort, anxiety or hanxious, panic, apathy
Energy	**Unpleasant:** Fatigue, *sleepiness*, feeling weak

Instead of...	Try this...
Skipping your lunch break and then being so hungry you stop at the drive-through instead of waiting to get home	Eating on your lunch break because it's the only chance you have to eat at work and it holds you over so you can eat dinner at home.
Skipping breakfast because you binged last night and now you're not hungry.	Eating breakfast, even if you don't feel hungry because you want to break the binge/restrict cycle.
Not eating all day because your meds zap your appetite and binge eating at night.	Eating every three to four hours so you don't binge eat at night.
Getting hyperfocused for 6+ hours and then bingeing.	Eating a snack because you know you are likely to get hyperfocused on work.

What are Your Hunger Cues?

Keep a list or pictures of hunger cues at your desk or on your fridge as a visual reminder as you build awareness of what hunger feels like in your body. (You are welcome to print any of my Instagram posts on hunger cues.) Other visual cues to remind yourself to check in with your body about hunger cues include leaving sticky notes on your bathroom mirror, on the door to your garage, or even making a screensaver for your phone.

used to consider eating for stimulation as part of emotional hunger because it can feel like boredom eating, eating to procrastinate, and/or eating for reward. But when I want to eat for stimulation it feels more like there's an itch in my brain that needs to be scratched rather than soothing an emotion, which usually shows up in my body.

Eating for stimulation can feel like needing to do something with your hands or your mouth. You might seek out specific tastes like sweet, spicy, salty, or sour. Or you might seek out specific textures like crunchy, chewy, or gummy. Like emotional hunger, brain hunger can lead to overeating or binge eating if food is your only tool for stimulation.

Like emotional hunger, it is okay to honor this form of hunger. Choosing not to because it's "bad" or because it's not a physical hunger cue may lead to not eating enough. We will dive deeper into eating for stimulation in chapter 6.

Taste Hunger

Taste hunger is wanting to eat something because it sounds yummy. Like many of my clients, you may be thinking that if you ate everything you thought was tasty, you'd never stop! But when you've made peace with food and your body learns it can have tasty food whenever you want it because it's no longer restricted, you won't feel the need to say yes every single time you see something delicious. Plus, you probably wouldn't feel great if you did.

Yes, it is okay to want and choose to eat something because it sounds tasty. If you are craving a specific taste or texture in your mouth, then that may be more brain hunger or seeking stimulation. I think of taste hunger as usually unplanned, like when a coworker brings in brownies and offers you one. You aren't hungry, but a gooey, chocolatey brownie sounds delicious so you say yes—and that's okay.

Barriers to Recognizing and Honoring Your Hunger

Now that you've learned about the different types of hunger, let's take a closer look at some things other than ADHD that can disrupt our ability to recognize our hunger cues. In chapter 4, we will discuss strategies for overcoming these barriers and how to set up a pattern of regular eating that works for you.

Chronic Restriction/Dieting

Dieting and chronic restriction can make hunger cues go mute. If you have a long history of dieting or restricting, your hunger cues may not be very reliable at first. Eating regularly can help wake up your hunger cues. It is also very common to feel significantly more hunger than usual when you get out of a period of restriction.

Diets often encourage "hacks" to try to suppress your appetite. A few examples include drinking lots of coffee, green tea, or diet soda, chewing gum, and filling up on volume foods. You may be tempted to try these things, but your body is biologically hardwired to ensure that you get the nourishment you need. The best way to keep your appetite in check is to make sure you are actually eating enough regularly throughout the day. In chapter 8, we will discuss how types of foods such as protein and fiber, can play a huge role in keeping your appetite in check.

Having the Right Mindset

Eating is an act of self-care. As one of our most basic human needs, eating is non-negotiable. Try to view taking time to eat on a regular basis as doing something for your future self. Talk to yourself as if you are talking to a younger version of you. How would you take care of a younger version of yourself if they were hungry?

Sickness

Sickness, whether it's an acute or chronic illness, can impact your appetite. Generally, you may not have the desire to eat or prepare food when you're sick. You may want to honor practical hunger or lean more on your safe foods, or foods that give a reliable sensory experience and provide comfort or a sense of safety, when you are not feeling well. If you don't eat while you are acutely sick, you will likely get a visit from the hunger monster when you start to feel better.

Stress

Everyone is different in terms of how their body responds to stress. You might be someone who gets hungrier when stressed. You might be someone who has zero appetite when stressed. Or you might be someone whose appetite is impacted depending on the source of the stress.

How does stress affect your appetite? Learning how to manage and decrease stressors in your life can have positive effects on your relationship with food, managing ADHD, and improving your overall quality of life.

Recognizing Bodily Cues When You Have ADHD: Fullness

Now that we've talked about how your body tells you it needs nourishment, let's talk about how it tells you that you're full. Fullness is your body's way of letting you know that it has enough food to do all the processes it needs to do to keep you alive and functioning. Eating past fullness means that you have eaten more than what your body needs in that moment, and you may temporarily feel uncomfortable.

Some people think if they eat past fullness, they are failing at Intuitive Eating. But I think what matters is whether you choose to do so or not. Binge eating can feel like an out-of-body experience that you cannot control. In Intuitive Eating, you have the autonomy to decide how much or little food is right for your body in that moment based on how hungry you are.

Physical Signs of Fullness

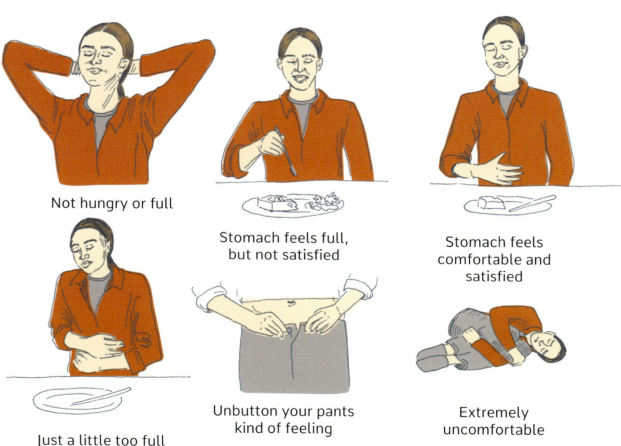

Not hungry or full

Stomach feels full, but not satisfied

Stomach feels comfortable and satisfied

Just a little too full

Unbutton your pants kind of feeling

Extremely uncomfortable

Signs of Fullness

Part of Body	Potential Fullness Cue
Head	**Pleasant:** fewer food-related thoughts, cravings feel satisfied, less interest in food, better focus on other things **Unpleasant:** so painfully full that you don't even want to think about food
Taste buds	**Unpleasant:** Food not as tasty as it was at the beginning of the meal or snack
Stomach	**Pleasant:** warm, some pressure or tightness, stomach more rounded and stretched (this is normal) **Unpleasant:** painfully full or bloated sensation in stomach area, nauseous or sick to stomach, uncomfortable tightness in midsection
Energy	**Pleasant:** may have more energy or feel a little bit of sleepiness **Unpleasant:** significant sleepiness
Mood	**Pleasant:** Shifts to feeling more pleasant, neutral, or relaxed

Signs of Fullness

Just like hunger, many ADHDers may not recognize fullness until it's in a more extreme form, which feels unpleasant and uncomfortable. Comfortable fullness can feel like a more neutral or even pleasant sensation. You no longer feel hungry and you don't feel too full, but if you were to keep eating a few more bites you'd start to feel uncomfortable.

Imagine a pendulum swinging from extreme hunger to extreme fullness. This is what happens when you go too long without eating or restrict your food. **If you wait until you're ravenous to eat, then you are more likely to eat until you're stuffed.** The only way to learn your fullness cues is to give yourself permission to eat enough.

Once you've learned your unique hunger cues, you'll find that your fullness cues will likely be the opposite. For example, if you get hangry when you're hungry, then you might notice that your mood shifts to feeling more pleasant or relaxed when you're full. If having trouble concentrating on your work is a hunger cue, you might notice that you are able to focus after eating.

The table above highlights some signs of fullness you may experience. Pleasant signs of fullness are signs of comfortable fullness. Unpleasant signs of fullness are usually a result of overeating and binge eating.

Barriers to Feeling Your Fullness

Distracted Eating

Every single client I have worked with finds it challenging to "eat mindfully," or eat without any distractions. I remember the first time I tried to eat this way; it was a nails-on-the-chalkboard kind of experience. I remember thinking, "People just sit here and eat?! How?! What the hell do they think about?!" I lasted all of five minutes before I put my headphones on to listen to music so I could finish my lunch.

However, being overly distracted while eating can also be a barrier to fullness. For some ADHDers, their brain doesn't retain the memory of eating as well when they are distracted. This makes it more likely that you'll forget you've eaten or how much you've eaten, which may result in overeating. Eating with distractions also disrupts the rewarding qualities of food, or the effects of dopamine. Not having this sense of reward may lead to eating more food.

In Intuitive Eating, you're encouraged to eat *mostly* distraction-free. Don't worry, I am not going to tell you that you need to eat this way. Instead, **the key is to find your Goldilocks zone: the level of sensory input that is just right for you.** This is especially important if you eat alone. Figure out how much and what kind of sensory input is most helpful so you can feel more present while eating.

A few examples are:

- Auditory Input: music, a podcast, audiobook, or mindful eating meditation. Another option is to eat your meal in a noisier public space, like a park or on your patio, instead of inside in a quiet space.
- Visual Input: TV shows, YouTube, people watching, etc.
- Tactile Input: having a fidget in one hand while you eat or rolling a tennis ball under your foot

Explore what works best for you. If you eat with distractions and still find yourself uncomfortably full afterward, you can also try the following strategies.

THREE-BITE CHECK-IN

If you know you are going to be distracted or doing other things while you eat, try a three-bite check-in. At the beginning, somewhere in the middle, and toward the end of the meal or snack, pause and check in. How is the food tasting and how is the texture? How does your stomach feel? Are you noticing any signs of fullness? If so, it might be time to stop eating.

START SMALL WITH A SNACK

If you do want to explore eating with fewer or no distractions, consider starting with a snack. Your brain may be more open to trying this with a snack because snacks tend to take less time to eat than a meal. Pay attention to the taste and texture of the food as you eat. Check in with your body periodically to see if you are starting to notice any signs of fullness.

Unhelpful Messages About Eating: The Clean Plate Club

If you are a member of the Clean Plate Club, then chances are your parents had rules that meant you needed to eat everything on your plate before you could get dessert or leave the table. Cleaning your plate as a child basically conditioned you to ignore your body's messages that you were full. Instead you may have routinely eaten beyond your stopping point.

Parents often instigate the Clean Plate Club with well-meaning intentions like wanting to make sure their kids are eating enough "healthy" foods. I remember my mom telling me, "You better eat your broccoli because there are starving kids in other countries." I responded by telling my mom that I would give them my food if I could because I was full. Kids are often better at listening to their bodies than adults.

What helped me unlearn this mindset was remembering that eating past fullness does far more damage to the body and mind than discarding or saving food for later. Now I have zero problem leaving two bites of food on my plate at home or at a restaurant, and neither should you.

The People You Eat With

Generally, the more people we eat with and the longer the meal, the more we eat. But I find for ADHDers, it also depends on how well we know the people, how comfortable we are around them, and what our eating environment is like.

If the people you eat with create a stressful eating environment, it can prevent you from feeling full or it can even zap your appetite. To avoid this, don't use mealtime as an opportunity to settle arguments—or at least wait until everyone has eaten before bringing up a topic that might start an argument. You may find comfort or safety in eating alone, and that is 100 percent fine. When I had coworkers, I preferred to eat alone so I could recharge my social battery.

Restriction or Food Rules

Metabolically, chronic restriction, especially dieting, can result in a decrease in your fullness hormone (leptin) and an increase in your hunger hormone (ghrelin). This can lead to never actually feeling full when you are dieting or trying to restrict. As discussed before, when you restrict what or how much you eat, you will never feel full and satiated.

Food Rules: Love or Control?

Food rules can be based in love or in control. You may have food restrictions due to food allergies or sensitivities. Choosing to avoid those foods because they make you sick or could kill you is a food rule rooted in a love for your body and your life. On the other hand, trying to avoid carbs because you are afraid they will make you gain weight is a rule based in control and fear. Food rules based in control or fear tend to backfire.

For neurodivergent folks, having flexible boundaries or guardrails when it comes to eating can be rules based in love—such as making sure you're eating a minimum amount of food at a meal so you know you're getting the nourishment you need.

If you have a history of dieting or restricting, you may need to challenge what constitutes a "serving" of food. Remember, serving sizes are not the recommended amount of that food, but rather, the average amount consumed of a food. You may need more than a serving of a particular food to feel full and that is okay.

Strategies for Achieving Lasting Fullness

Eat a Combination of Macronutrients

We will be discussing this in much more depth in chapter 9, but all three macronutrients—high-fiber carbohydrates, fats, and proteins—play a role in helping you feel full longer (unlike simple carbs, which wear off more quickly). Each macronutrient is a key piece in the puzzle of lasting fullness.

At meals, try including a food from each of these categories. For example: chicken breast (protein) with roasted potatoes (fiber), and asparagus (fiber) tossed in olive oil (fat). With snacks, aim for at least two of the three macronutrients to help you stay fuller for longer. For example, pineapple (fiber) and cottage cheese (protein). If you don't include a combination of macronutrients, you'll feel hungrier sooner.

"Dress Up" Air-Foods & Volume Foods

Examples of air-foods are rice cakes, 100-calorie snack packs, and popcorn. Volume foods include fruits and non-starchy veggies.

Both air-foods and volume foods fill you up but do not provide you with a feeling of lasting fullness. That doesn't mean you need to avoid them. Instead, think about how you can "dress them up" with protein and/or fat so you can stay full for longer.

Volume foods, particularly fruits and non-starchy veggies, have health-promoting and disease-preventing benefits, but even if you eat a lot of them on their own, you will probably not feel full for very long. Pair them with a source of fat and/or protein to help you feel full for longer. Consider:

- Pretzels vs. pretzels + hummus
- Popcorn vs. popcorn + mixed nuts
- Apple vs. apple + cheese
- Strawberries vs. strawberries + low-fat Greek yogurt
- Carrots vs. carrots + ranch

Don't get me wrong, I really enjoy pretzels and chips, but if I only eat pretzels or chips, I need A LOT of them to feel satisfied. **Pairing carb-based snacks with fat and/or protein means you still get to enjoy your favorite snacks.** Does that mean you need to do this every time you have them? Absolutely not. But if you find you could eat a whole bag of potato chips before you realize you're full, pairing them with a fat or protein might be helpful.

The Connection Between Satisfaction and Fullness

Satisfaction is a key to honoring fullness and important enough that it has its own principle in Intuitive Eating. Satisfaction plays a big role in being able to stop eating when you're physically full. Does this mean every single meal and snack you eat needs to be the most satisfying, delicious thing you've ever had? No.

Most of us do not have the ability or the money to eat whatever appeals most to us on demand. While you should try to include foods that satisfy you in most meals and snacks, sometimes a meal you prepare or order out just doesn't quite hit the spot. When this happens, you can choose something else that does or remind yourself that a more satisfying eating experience will happen in the future.

What happens when you overlook the satisfaction factor and deny yourself what you really want to eat? Imagine you are on a diet and craving a cookie. But cookies are off-limits on this diet, so you decide to have some strawberries with some sugar-free whipped cream instead. But you aren't satisfied and all you can think about is having a cookie.

You scour through the pantry for a "healthier" option and find chocolate chips. You promise yourself that you'll only have one serving and put the package away. But it wasn't enough, so you grab a few more and a few more after that until you've had half the bag. When you realize you "blew" your diet, you say screw it, and go on to finish the chocolate chips and proceed to eat a dozen cookies you got delivered.

Afterward, you spend the evening flooded with guilt and beat yourself up for not having any willpower. Why didn't you just have the strawberries and sugar-free whipped cream? It should have been enough, but it wasn't what your body actually wanted. Now, you feel uncomfortably full and vow to do better tomorrow. Sound familiar?

If you listen, your body will let you know what it needs. Not honoring a craving sets you up to chase or eat around that craving. In the above example, if you would've just eaten the cookies to begin with, even if you ate the same amount of them, it still would have been less food. The big takeaway here is that if you are craving a cookie, it is very unlikely that strawberries are going to satisfy you—so give yourself permission to eat the cookie!

Tracking Hunger and Fullness and Why It Can Help

Tracking your hunger and fullness can be helpful for some folks. If you are moving away from counting calories or macros, tracking your hunger and fullness can give you different information that can help you learn to listen and trust your body to tell you how much to eat. If you have a history of eating disorders or disordered eating, this may be triggering for you. If so, I would just focus on eating every three to four hours and include certain foods at each meal and snack.

Hunger/Fullness Scale

The hunger/fullness scale is one tool often used in IE that rates your hunger/fullness on a scale of 1 to 10. Many ADHDers, myself included, don't find this tool particularly helpful, and that's okay. Ideally, you want to try to eat when you are at a 3 or a 4 on the hunger/fullness scale and you want to stop eating around a 6 or a 7. This prevents you from getting overly hungry and overly full. So basically, you want to stay in the middle of the hunger scale. If you drop to a 0 or 1, it's likely that you'll bounce back by overeating to a 9 or a 10 on the hunger/fullness scale.

An alternative to rating your hunger/fullness on a scale of 1 to 10 is to rate the quality of your hunger/fullness as pleasant, unpleasant, and neutral. I find this more useful, especially if it's hard for you to determine if you are a 3 hungry or 4 hungry. For me, unpleasant is when the hunger monster shows up or when I'm stuffed from eating too much. Pleasant hunger/fullness is when I eat when I feel hungry and stop when I am comfortably full. Neutral would be when I am honoring practical hunger.

Sensory Specific Satiety

Sensory specific satiety is using your senses to help you determine when you are comfortably full. This is when your taste buds start to become desensitized to the taste. You may notice this before you start to feel full. I think of this as like a flashing yellow light warning you to pause and check in with your body. You may want to wait a few minutes to see if fullness emerges. Other signs of sensory specific satiety include when the texture and appearance of the food is no longer appealing and you can no longer smell the food.

Stopping When You Are No Longer Hungry vs. When You Feel Full

You may want to pause when you no longer feel hungry instead of when you start to feel full. The sensations of fullness can take a little time to emerge after eating. If you stop when you feel full, then you are more likely to eat past comfortable fullness. If you are a fast eater, you may want to hit the pause button before you decide to get more food to give your stomach a chance to communicate to your brain that you are full.

Exercises to Improve Interoceptive Awareness

Even though we have differences in interoceptive awareness, it doesn't mean it's something we can't strengthen or improve. Here are some tools and exercises you can use to improve interoceptive awareness.

Mindfulness Practices

Mindfulness practices can be extremely helpful to build better mind-body connection and to cultivate better physical and emotional control over how your body responds to stress and distress. These practices can help you with self-regulation so you stop turning to food.

- **Meditation:** Meditation can be hard for some ADHDers. Often it's about finding the meditation approach that's right for you. The first meditation practice I learned was supposed to be done two times a day for 45 minutes each time. This didn't work for me. But I discovered I can do a 5- to 15-minute Headspace Meditation instead of scrolling or being on my phone when I return from my daily walk. Other apps include Insight Timer, Calm, and The Mindfulness App.
- **Body Scan:** Most body scans require you to sit still or lie down and scan your body from your head to your toes. But being still and relaxed is not natural for ADHDers. Instead, Kelly Mahler, an occupational therapist specializing in interoception, recommends a more active, playful approach to connect and engage with your body. You can start a body scan while you cook, dance, shower, or cuddle with your dog. See the appendix for more resources.
- **Somatic Exercises:** Yoga, dance, and tai chi are a few forms of movement that can help improve the mind-body connection. These exercises are ways to engage in mindfulness through movement. For example, when you do yoga, you focus on your body and how flowing through different postures makes you feel. You also learn to regulate your breathing and how it feels to tense and relax parts of your body.

Body Check-In

If you don't feel ready to try any of the previous practices, then try setting an alarm twice a day that's labeled "What do I need?" You can set this alarm on your phone, Google calendar, smart watch, or any other device you use to remind yourself to do something.

For many of my clients, they are so focused on getting their work tasks or other projects done that they forget to check in with themselves. This open-ended question only takes a few seconds but it's important. You may find your body needs food, water, a stretch break, or to use the bathroom. Eventually, you may not need the alarm or reminder because checking in with your body will become a natural practice. In the next chapter, we will explore other ways to use alarms to help you eat more consistently.

Finding Extra Help and Support

If interoception is something you really struggle with, then you might need some additional external support to remind you to eat or just check in with your body. And, if being present in your physical body is dysregulating or triggering due to a history of trauma, I recommend working with a trauma-informed therapist. They will be able to help create a safe environment and support you as you relearn how to be in your physical body.

CHAPTER 4

ADHDers are Consistently Inconsistent . . . Including with Food

"Chaotic," "inconsistent," or "all over the place" are common phrases my clients use to describe their eating patterns. You may have days where it feels as if all you do is eat and then other days when food barely crosses your mind. In the previous chapter, we discussed how to listen to your body so you can nourish it. In this chapter, we will discuss how to work through barriers and how to set up a pattern of eating that works with your ADHD brain. If you're a Binge/Restrictor or a Grazer, this chapter will hopefully be helpful for you.

What, When, and How Will You Eat?

Before you focus on the "what" aspect of eating (as in "What am I going to eat?"), you need to focus on the "when" and "how." When it comes to managing ADHD nutrition, many people get hung up on what they are going to eat and skip over when and how they are going to eat. A house needs a strong foundation to withstand the weather. Your eating pattern is the foundation that enables you to handle the stress that life throws your way. Unsurprisingly, it's easier to do things when you aren't hungry.

ADHD expert Dr. Edward Hallowell describes ADHDers as consistently inconsistent. This description applies to our eating patterns too. I eat about every three to four hours (although there are times when I'm hyperfocused that I stretch this), but I don't have scheduled mealtimes.

The way I feed myself also changes depending on the season of life I am in. For example, while writing this book I've outsourced more by ordering grocery delivery, using meal kit

delivery, and eating more frozen meals because I don't have the spoons to put toward cooking. When this book is done and I have more free time, I will likely go back to grocery shopping myself and doing more cooking. But for ADHDers, the goal is to eat more consistently at a frequency that helps your body feel safe, energized, and nourished. This does not mean we have to be robots and eat at the same time every single day (although if that works for you, that's great). By eating consistently, we can stop the pendulum from swinging back and forth between eating nothing and bingeing.

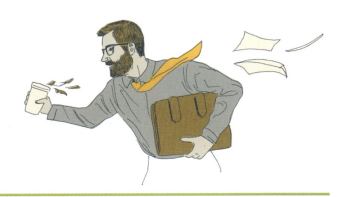

Common Inconsistent Eating Patterns for ADHDers

There are two common eating patterns I see with my clients that relate to inconsistency. The first eating pattern is exemplified by the Grazer eating profile from chapter 1. This type of ADHDer doesn't really have a plan when it comes to their eating. At work they stop by the break room or their coworker's desk for a snack. They stop at the drive-through on their way home because they didn't plan ahead for dinner. If they work from home, any trip to the kitchen results in a handful of something from the pantry or fridge.

If this is you, you probably don't know what hunger feels like because you never really let yourself go long enough without eating or drinking to feel hunger pangs. You may still binge eat, especially as a reward, a way to procrastinate on a task, or just because you were bored.

The second eating pattern revolves around the Binge/Restrictor eating profile. This cycle usually involves not eating enough during the day or eating inconsistently, which leads to insatiable hunger and binge eating at night. This cycle can happen with or without meds, but, as we learned in chapter 1, meds make it a lot easier to get stuck in this cycle.

ADHD Binge/Restrict Cycle

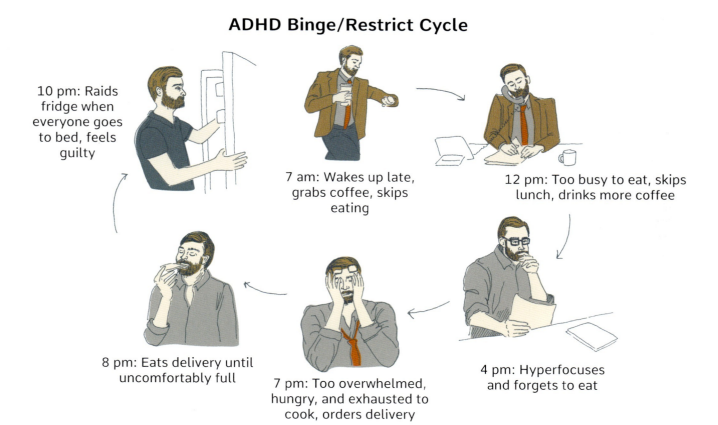

10 pm: Raids fridge when everyone goes to bed, feels guilty

7 am: Wakes up late, grabs coffee, skips eating

12 pm: Too busy to eat, skips lunch, drinks more coffee

8 pm: Eats delivery until uncomfortably full

7 pm: Too overwhelmed, hungry, and exhausted to cook, orders delivery

4 pm: Hyperfocuses and forgets to eat

These two eating patterns are two sides of the same coin. A Grazer is always eating regardless of their hunger and the Binge/Restrictor is often not eating (at least during the day) regardless of their hunger. Both can benefit from creating a flexible structure around eating.

The goal of establishing an eating pattern is not to make you eat like a neurotypical person. The goal is to bring some stability and predictability to eating patterns and remove the chaos around food. This doesn't mean that you have to eat at the exact same time every single day. Having a general guide around *when* you will eat frees up brain space to figure out *what* to eat.

Why Is It So Difficult for ADHDers to Eat Consistently?

When trying to make behavior changes with ADHD, I find it extremely helpful to understand what barriers exist to implementing change. Just knowing that eating more consistently can be helpful doesn't always translate to doing it. Digging into why it's difficult to do something when you have ADHD can help you uncover solutions and get over the barriers that are preventing action. There are several reasons ADHDers find it challenging to eat consistently.

Differences in Interoceptive Awareness

Last chapter, we covered how differences in interoception can make it harder to recognize when you're hungry and full. These differences may lead to forgetting to eat, eating when you aren't really hungry, etc. In this chapter, we will explore external supports or accommodations you can make to ensure you get enough food if your body is not a reliable way to determine if you are hungry.

ADHD Meds

ADHD meds add an extra layer on top of standard ADHD interoception differences that can make it more challenging to recognize when you are hungry. Meds often fuel the ADHD binge/restrict cycle. It can be challenging to eat regularly throughout the day when you don't get the same cues to remind you to eat as a neurotypical person.

No Structure

If you are either the Grazer or the Binge/Restrictor, then you might not ever have much structure around eating. The section with meal patterns in this chapter can help you find a way to create an eating structure that works best for you.

Hyperfocus and Time Blindness

Dr. Russell Barkley, a psychologist and ADHD researcher, describes ADHDers perception of time as either "now" or "not now." When you aren't hungry, it's "not now," so you don't think about food until you are in the "now," or ravenous. When you're hyperfocused, hours can feel like minutes. You may recognize a hunger cue but don't do anything about it. I like to think of it like a blip on the radar. You notice it, but it disappears before you can process and react to it.

One of my clients was frustrated that she was bingeing at night because she thought she was "eating enough and regularly" during the day.

But she ate breakfast around 7:00 am, lunch around 11:00 am, and then wouldn't eat again until 6:00 or 7:00 at night. When she got home, she'd binge eat snacks because she was too hungry to cook a meal.

Through our work, this client realized that what felt like four hours was actually more like seven hours without eating! She decided to pack two extra snacks and set alarms at 2:00 pm and at 5:00 pm to remind herself to eat. Adding the snacks into her schedule meant she wasn't so ravenous when she got home from work. She was able to actually cook dinner instead of raiding the pantry.

The Benefits of Eating Regularly

Eating regularly is a tool for managing your ADHD because it helps keep your energy and blood sugar stable, gives your brain the fuel it needs to function, and regulates your mood. I know it can be difficult to make changes in how you do things, but believe me, getting in the habit of eating regularly is well worth it.

Stable Energy and Blood Sugar Levels

When your eating patterns are all over the place, so is your energy and your blood sugar levels. When you go for long periods of time without eating and then suddenly feel ravenous, you probably reach for quick sources of energy like chips or sweets or other simple carbs. These types of foods can quickly elevate your blood sugar levels. Dramatic fluctuations in blood sugar can make your ADHD traits more notice-able, especially inattentiveness, hyperactivity, and impulsivity. Eating regularly throughout the day is a way to give your body and brain a steady source of energy and nutrition.

Emotional Regulation

The longer you go without eating, the less stable your mood. Anyone with ADHD is going to experience emotional dysregulation. But it's a lot easier to have an ADHD negative spiral when you've barely eaten all day. Think about when you get really hungry. Aren't you more easily irritated, anxious, or overwhelmed? Our executive functions, one of which is regulating our emotions, simply don't work as well when we are hungry.

Ability to Make Intentional Food Choices

Executive function plays a role in decision-making, which is more challenging when you're ravenous. When you've reached this point, your body wants the quickest, fastest source of energy. This usually means simple carbs like chips, candy, soda, etc. These foods are tasty but not very filling, so you often need to eat a large amount to feel full.

Constantly reaching for these foods instead of more nutrient-dense options probably doesn't make you feel great physically or mentally. Many of my clients feel guilt or regret because they would have made a different choice if they weren't so hungry. Remember, this is your body trying to protect you and get you the energy it needs.

How to Establish a Regular Eating Pattern

I highly recommend establishing some sort of eating pattern so that you eat enough throughout the day. This is especially important if you want to stop binge eating at night. Eating regularly doesn't have to be the traditional meal pattern that includes three meals, a mid-morning snack, and a mid-afternoon snack. I invite you to explore different eating patterns to find the one that works best for you and feels sustainable.

Think of establishing a meal pattern as creating the scaffolding for eating regularly. Having some predetermined times for eating means you don't have to think about when to eat. It takes the guesswork out of it.

Which eating pattern you choose depends on your work and home life. For example, if you work 10- to 12-hour shifts, then you might have an eating pattern that you follow on your workdays and a different eating pattern on your days off. You are allowed to be flexible and adapt your eating to your schedule.

Practical hunger can play a big role in establishing a regular eating pattern. For example, you may not be hungry on your 30-minute lunch break, but you choose to honor practical hunger by eating so you don't end up ravenous and raiding your pantry or stopping through the fast-food drive-through on the way home. You might also honor practical hunger when your kids are napping or when you're between meetings.

You don't have to follow society's ideas of what the "right" time is for a meal. Mealtimes are a social construct. You are not a failure for eating lunch at say, 11:30 am instead of noon or dinner at 8:00 pm instead of 6:00 pm. It's fine to establish a meal pattern by setting more general time frames for when you eat certain meals or snacks. (Contrary to what a lot of diet influencers would have you believe, eating past 7:00 pm doesn't lead to automatic weight gain.)

All of the suggested meal patterns below encourage you to eat every three to four hours or five to six times per day. It's a good idea to eat something within the first hour or two of waking up and then every three to four hours until you go to bed. You may want to avoid eating an hour or two before bed, especially if you have acid reflux.

Meal Pattern 1: Traditional Meal Pattern

If you look up meal plans online or have worked with a dietitian in the past, then you're probably familiar with this eating pattern. In my opinion, the traditional meal pattern is ideal for ADHDers who work a more traditional nine-to-five type of job or follow this sort of schedule. This meal pattern may or may not include an evening snack after dinner.

Sample traditional meal pattern:

- Breakfast (7:00 am): 2 scrambled eggs + 2 slices of whole wheat toast + ½ avocado mashed on toast + blueberries
- Snack (10:00 am): cheese + nuts + dried fruit
- Lunch (1:00 pm): BLT + fruit salad + pickle + cookie
- Snack (4:00 pm): protein shake
- Dinner (7:00 pm): protein pasta + meat sauce + broccoli
- Optional Snack (9:00 pm): 2 cookies + glass of skim milk

Meal Pattern 2: Anchor Meals

If your ADHD meds zap your appetite, then you may want to explore the anchor meal pattern. With this meal pattern, your largest meals would be breakfast and dinner. Instead of having a more traditional-sized lunch, you have three to four snacks or mini meals during the day. This can work well because your appetite will likely be strongest in the morning before you take your meds and in the evening when they wear off. The downside to this eating pattern is that you may need to eat more often.

Sample anchor meal pattern:

- Breakfast (7:00 am): Breakfast burrito + bell pepper slices + coffee
- Snack (10:00 am): apple + cheese stick
- Snack (1:00 pm): Greek yogurt + berries + walnuts
- Snack (4:00 pm): carrots + single-serving cup of hummus + protein drink
- Dinner (7:00 pm): grilled chicken tenders + baked potato + side salad + cookie

Meal Pattern 3: Flip-Flop Meal Pattern

The flip-flop meal pattern is ideal for ADHDers who struggle with eating breakfast. For this meal pattern, you flip your breakfast and mid-morning snack. You could also flip other meals or snacks if that makes more sense for you.

Sample flip-flop meal pattern:

- Snack (7:00 am): coffee + a scoop of protein powder
- Breakfast (9:00 am): 2 egg bites + banana
- Lunch (12:00 pm): Mediterranean salad kit + grilled chicken + salad dressing + whole wheat pita bread + square of dark chocolate
- Snack (3:00 pm): sliced bell peppers + single-serving cup of guacamole
- Dinner (7:00 pm): tofu veggie stir-fry + rice
- Optional snack (9:00 pm): strawberries + almonds

How Can I Work with My ADHD Brain to Eat Regularly?

Now that we've discussed some sample meal patterns, let's discuss how you can make them happen. In this section, I will cover some tools and strategies that have helped me and my clients eat enough, regularly, by adding flexible structure to the day and helping you remember to eat. Before I dive in, you may want to reflect on what tools or strategies help you remember to do other daily tasks or activities. Can you use any of those tools or strategies to support you in eating every three to four hours?

Adopt the "Fed Is Best" Mindset

"Fed is best" or "Eating something is better than nothing" are two common mantras that my clients find helpful when it comes to eating regularly. If you are a perfectionist or fad dieter, you might skip a meal or snack because the only option is a "bad" option. But this sets you up to get overly hungry and binge later. The fed is best mindset can help you unlearn the "good" vs. "bad" food mindset and adopt a more neutral approach.

I'll be honest that it may feel like a chore to eat more regularly during the day at first. Remember that eating is an act of self-care. Every time you choose to pause so you can eat, you are engaging in self-care. Eating is an opportunity to not only connect with yourself, but if you eat with other people, it's also a chance to connect with others.

You can change your perspective on eating regularly and your mindset. For example, you might view eating a snack as a way to help transition from one task to another. Or you could view your lunch as a break from the grind and an opportunity to fill up your executive function battery so you can get through the rest of the day.

Find Time Where You Think You Have None

You may feel as if you do not have time to eat. Or maybe you don't know how to make time to eat. If, for example, you can't take an hour lunch, then intentionally carving out 15 minutes may feel more manageable. You'll still be making a commitment to eating regularly. This will make it easier to remember, and you'll be less likely to skip a meal.

It may seem obvious, but eating does take time. You are not being selfish, unproductive, or an inconvenience when you pause to nourish your body and brain. If anything, making time to eat will help your meds work more effectively and give you the energy you need to work through your to-do list.

Making time to nourish your body is a way to show it you respect and care about it.

I guarantee that if you explore your day-to-day schedule, you can find pockets of time to eat.

Pull up your Google calendar, take out your half-used planner, or find a week-at-a-glance calendar that breaks days down by the hour. Set a timer for 20 to 30 minutes. Now, write out a typical schedule for each day of the week, noting any pockets of time when you could eat. Be honest with yourself. Include how much time you spend doomscrolling, watching TV, playing video games, etc. Can any of these activities be cut back to give yourself time to eat?

If you're still struggling to make time for eating, consider this: Are you able to make time for your boss or coworker when they add an appointment to your calendar? If so, could you create a standing meeting with yourself everyday so that you have 20 minutes blocked off on your schedule for lunch?

Other Strategies to Make Eating More Consistent

Strategies like reminders are helpful for ADHDers because they help externalize some of our executive function. Here are some examples.

Use Alarms

Sometimes ADHDers skip meals because they literally forget to eat. If this is you, alarms can be a great tool to help you get used to eating regularly and help with time blindness. (Not every ADHDer finds alarms helpful. If you don't, feel free to skip this section.)

You can use your phone, smart watch, laptop, or smart home device to set your alarms. The alarm my clients have found the most helpful is an alarm labeled "What do I need?" This kind of alarm can help you practice checking in with yourself. See chapter 3 for more info about this.

Here are a few tips to make alarms work for you:

- Label your alarms so you know what they are for.
- Designate a sound for alarms that remind you to eat.
- Use a stand-alone alarm (i.e., not your phone), so you have to get up to turn it off.
- Set a follow-up alarm, one to remind you when you have something to do and another one as a follow-up.
- Use suggestive language. If you don't like demands, consider phrases like "Are you hungry?" "Do you want to eat lunch soon?" "Would you like to take a break and grab a snack?"

Pair Eating with Another Activity

Some ADHDers find it helpful to pair activities together to remember to do them. For example, I pair breakfast and lunch with taking my morning and afternoon ADHD meds. This is when my appetite will be at its best, which makes it easier to eat. It also helps remind me to eat and take my ADHD meds, which is helpful because if I take my ADHD meds too late in the day, I won't be able to sleep at night.

My one caveat here is to avoid pairing eating with overly distracting activities that make it hard for you to check in with your hunger/fullness cues or make you forget to eat. These might include scrolling social media or binge watching your favorite TV show.

Activities to pair with eating:

- Taking ADHD meds, especially if you take short-acting meds twice per day.
- Feeding your kids or pets.
- Drinking water.
- Work breaks or transitions from one task to another.

Body Doubling

Body doubling can be useful if you don't like eating alone. You could join a virtual body doubling group and FaceTime or Zoom with a friend while you cook or eat. Or ask a coworker or partner to eat with you during lunch.

Visual Cues

If out of sight, out of mind rings true for you, then you might want to consider visual cues. Consider where you might need visual cues, such as in your office, kitchen, or car. Some of my clients will keep shelf-stable snacks in a bin or a desk drawer. You might keep some snacks on your counter to remind you to eat or store snacks at eye level in your refrigerator or pantry. You could leave snacks or water bottles in your car, though I probably wouldn't do this when it is hot outside.

External Support

If remembering to eat is a big challenge, you may want to consider asking your partner, friend, sibling, or coworker if they can support you with a gentle reminder to eat. Get their permission and talk about how they can show up for you in this way. If you have an ADHD buddy who struggles with this, consider leaning on each other.

One of my clients tries to work through lunch. Her boss knows that she has a complicated relationship with food, so she and her coworkers remind her to take a lunch break. Getting a text from a friend with a photo of a lunch meal with the caption: "Eating this yummy burrito bowl for lunch. What are you having for lunch today?" is also a good reminder. My partner regularly makes me some food when he prepares a meal. This way when I have a busy workday, the food is ready.

Automate Your Eating

During my workweek, I have some predetermined meals and snacks that I eat regularly. If I had to guess, I eat the same snacks about 70 percent of the time. This makes it easier for me to honor my hunger on meds and means I have fewer choices to make during the day. (I will eat a different snack if I'm really in the mood for it.) If eating while on meds is challenging, try to find a few options that you can tolerate, and prioritize always having them around. If you need to, get a subscription and have the snacks shipped to your house to make sure you always have them on hand.

Eat Breakfast

Breakfast simply means "breaking the fast," and it's important to eat it whether you take meds or not. If you take meds, do so with a meal that's high in protein. If you want to stop binge eating at night, you need to fill yourself up earlier in the day. Skipping breakfast, whether intentional or unintentional, keeps you trapped in the ADHD binge/restrict cycle. Breakfast doesn't have to be traditional "breakfast" foods like eggs, cereal, bacon, or oatmeal. It can be something like leftover chicken stir-fry or a PB&J sandwich with fruit.

Tips for Eating Consistently While on Stimulants

As we mentioned in chapter 3, ADHD meds can make it more challenging to honor your hunger because they can suppress your appetite. The effect is typically the strongest when you start ADHD meds, depending on the dose. Over time, your body will get more adjusted to the appetite-suppressing effect. So if you really aren't hungry at first, give it some time.

My biggest tip when starting ADHD meds is to prioritize practical hunger and get into an eating routine. This may mean eating something every three to four hours, even if it's a small amount of food.

Remember, eating is a priority, even if your brain says otherwise. Not having an appetite is not "good." Not eating on your meds will likely set you up to binge when they wear off at night. Going all day without eating will also negatively impact your mental and physical health. Remember, these meds aren't weight loss tools or designed to restrict intentionally. Even with Vyvanse, a medication approved for ADHD and binge eating disorder, you still need to eat food when you take it.

If you don't eat enough on your meds, you will need to prepare yourself for the hunger monster to show up at night when they wear off. Remember, there is nothing wrong with you if the hunger monster shows up. It's trying to protect you from getting malnourished!

ADHD meds are like the grease that helps the engine run smoothly. Food is like the fuel that gets you from point A to point B. We need both to function.

Aim to eat about every three to four hours. If you don't want to use time, aim for eating five to six times per day. If you miss a snack, that's okay. This does not have to be perfect. The more you do this, the more your body will start to expect food around those times.

What Can I Eat When My Meds Make Eating Gross?

No one wants to force themselves to eat when medication makes food unappealing or even grosses them out. But just like exploring non-traditional eating patterns to get into a routine of eating regularly, you might need to find some foods that you can tolerate eating. Keep the following types of foods on hand to make it easier to eat while you are medicated or for those times when executive function challenges make feeding yourself difficult.

Nutrient-Dense Liquids

On or off meds, liquids can be a great option if solid food sounds unappealing or you don't have time to stop and eat. Some examples of liquids include protein shakes, drinkable yogurts, soups, smoothies, etc.

This may require you to challenge the diet culture belief that it's "bad" to drink your calories. Does that mean you should live on soda because your meds suppress your appetite? No. It won't make you feel good and it's not great for your health in the long-term. But for folks who struggle with eating (due to meds or otherwise), nutrient-dense liquids can make the difference in getting nourishment or not.

If you know liquids will be a frequent part of your eating pattern, choose liquids that provide more than just added sugar. Sugar-sweetened beverages, particularly soda and energy drinks, are delicious and fun, but they provide very little nutrition outside of calories or energy. Prioritize having nutrient-dense options on hand so that it is an accessible option.

"Kid" Foods or Beige Foods

Yes, adults can eat "kid" foods. It doesn't make you any less of an adult. It just means you are ensuring you are fed and honoring your sensory preferences. If someone shames you for it, send them my way. "Kid" foods are often safe foods, especially for folks with sensory sensitivities, which we will chat more about in chapter 7.

Kid foods are predictable in terms of taste, texture, and aroma. Many of them tend to be softer in texture, blander in taste, and beige in color. They often are easier to prepare or require fewer spoons. They may be nostalgic foods or comfort foods. They also may be less expensive. Common foods in this category include chicken nuggets, french fries, mashed potatoes, mac and cheese, grilled cheese, PB&J sandwiches, instant ramen, potato chips, mozzarella sticks, cheese pizza, toast, pancakes, etc.

Ready-to-Eat Foods

Yes, it's okay to eat processed foods. These foods reduce the barrier to eating. If getting the big container of yogurt out of the fridge, finding a clean bowl and spoon, scooping it out, putting the yogurt back in the fridge, and then washing the dishes means you never eat your yogurt, then buy the individual yogurt cups. You'll actually eat it. It's okay to work smarter, not harder.

Yes, these may use more plastic. I totally understand the desire to live a more sustainable life, but if you are not eating consistently, have low energy, don't have enough spoons to prep food (which is 1000 percent okay), then consider making an accommodation for yourself. **Eating is a basic human need that you need to fulfill so you can show up as the best version of yourself.** And it's going to be really hard to help save the planet if you're running on empty all the time. You can always recycle or upcycle the plastic, whenever possible.

Eating enough, regularly, is the foundation not only to feeding yourself but also to using food as a part of how you manage your ADHD. When you find an eating pattern that works for you, life is sure to get in the way. This means you often can't do it perfectly, and that's part of being human. It doesn't mean that you need to scrap it. Overtime, as you allow yourself to use this eating pattern and other strategies to create a flexible structure, it will remove the chaos and feelings of being overwhelmed from your eating. Now that you've learned about why it's important to eat consistently, in the next chapter I'll explain why you might turn to food when you aren't hungry and what you can do about it.

CHAPTER 5

Why Am I Such an Emotional Eater?

Earlier, we discussed how binge eating is a response to restriction or an unmet need. One of those unmet needs can be our emotions. Since emotional dysregulation is a core feature of ADHD, it makes sense that ADHDers are more likely to emotionally eat. When you do not create space to feel and process your emotions, there's a good chance you will turn to less helpful coping strategies like food, alcohol, or online shopping.

Not all of us were taught how to feel our feelings as children. Some of us weren't raised in a home where it felt safe to do so. In those cases, food may have been the only coping tool available, and it still could be. If that's you, know that you're allowed to have feelings and your feelings are valid. It's essential to learn to feel your feelings so that you can decide what you like and what you don't, make good decisions, and pursue goals and dreams that are meaningful to you. This is especially important if you have ADHD because of the unique challenges we face.

Diet culture has created the false belief that all forms of emotional eating are bad. This is simply not true. Sometimes food is what you need or the only tool you have access to, and that's okay. I think of eating for emotional reasons to be like taking a cough drop for a sore throat. It may help alleviate some of the discomfort that you are feeling, but it is not going to fix or resolve whatever emotions triggered you to turn to food. You don't use cough drops when you are sick because you think they will cure your sore throat. You use them so you can get some relief.

Emotions vs. Feelings

Emotions and feelings are words that are often used interchangeably, but they are actually two different things. Emotions are automatic and unconscious responses. They are objective physiological reactions to a specific event like getting butterflies in your stomach when you see your crush or a racing heartbeat before you give a speech. They tend to be more intense and short-lived. Understanding the physical sensations that come from your body when you experience an emotion can help you become better at managing them. The six universal emotions are fear, anger, joy, sadness, disgust, and surprise.

Feelings are your interpretation of an experience. They may stem from emotions and are influenced by individual experiences (thoughts and memories), social norms, and culture. They tend to stick around longer than emotions and are more subjective. Unlike emotions, which can be seen through expressions, feelings can be hidden.

The goal is not to eliminate eating for emotional reasons. The goal is to acknowledge that eating may temporarily help, but it's not a solution for the things that are causing you to feel that way. It's also acknowledging that *for the most part* you will use other tools to cope with your feelings. If you do choose to eat for emotional reasons, it's an intentional and mindful experience, instead of an urgent and chaotic one. It's neutral. It's not dissociating or numbing with food.

In this chapter, we'll explore what emotional dysregulation is, how interoception plays a role in our emotions, identify emotional eating triggers, and learn how to build an emotional coping toolkit.

The Challenge of Emotional Dysregulation

Emotional dysregulation is a core feature and one of the biggest challenges of living with ADHD. While it is not in the DSM-5, most experts in the ADHD space agree that this is a key piece of living with ADHD. A 2020 study found that emotional dysregulation is correlated to the severity of ADHD traits in adults.

Often, emotional dysregulation can look like emotional overreaction, meaning how you feel does not match up with the cause of the feeling. This can show up as irritability, a short temper, or becoming overexcited or anxious about something.

It can be challenging to calm down when an emotion takes hold, which may be why ADHDers try to avoid feeling their feelings at all costs. Your big emotions may have led to people telling you that you are "too sensitive," "overly dramatic," or "too much." You may be more sensitive to rejection, disapproval, or even perceived rejection or disapproval. (This is sometimes referred to as rejection sensitive dysphoria.)

It's okay to have emotions, even big emotions. It's okay to feel your feelings. It's okay be sensitive. It's okay to safely express how you are feeling. Above all, remember: **You are not your emotions. You experience emotions.** Both good and bad emotions are a part of existing. While there may be emotions that are more pleasant and enjoyable, I find it helpful to view emotions in a neutral light.

How Being Emotionally Dysregulated Leads to Emotional Eating

In the last chapter, you learned how inconsistent eating patterns or not eating enough during the day can lead you to fall into the ADHD binge/restrict cycle. Both of these things can also make it easier to get emotionally dysregulated. This, in turn, may cause you to turn to food to regulate your emotions, hence "emotional eating." Food provides your brain with "feel good" neurotransmitters, such as

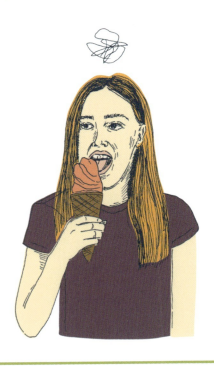

dopamine and serotonin, so you feel a sense of pleasure or calm. But relying on food as your go-to for emotional regulation will likely contribute to overeating or binge eating. In this chapter, we will discuss how to expand your tool kit so food is not your only option.

Is It Emotional Eating? Or a Reaction to Food Restriction and Dieting?

It can be difficult to know if you are eating for emotional reasons, to satisfy cravings, or to feel full as the result of restricting or dieting. It's a fact that if your tank is empty and you eat inconsistently, you are going to experience more emotional dysregulation and emotional hunger. When you combine feeling ravenous with feeling emotionally dysregulated, you have the perfect recipe for overeating or binge eating. In that moment, these are the only ways to get your body the energy it needs and get your brain the neurotransmitters it needs.

If there is an intense emotion or discomfort that accompanies your craving, then your emotions could be playing a bigger role. However, if no foods are off limits and you don't engage in physical or mental restriction, then you will not have the same intense cravings that happen when you are emotionally dysregulated and in a deprivation state.

When Emotional Eating Becomes Binge Eating

One big thing I have noticed while working with ADHDers who binge eat for emotional reasons is that food becomes a way to distract ourselves from working through our feelings. When we do this, the discomfort of being uncomfortably full and the shame for "being so out of control" or eating "bad" foods becomes the focus, instead of whatever deeper feeling we're experiencing. We end up burying our feelings so that we never actually work through them.

Would I Benefit from Therapy?

Therapy is an excellent tool for improving your ability to process and regulate your emotions. ADHDers can really benefit from having a safe place to process their feelings with someone who can be objective. Therapy can also be a great place to process your diagnosis and grieve the life you could've had if you had been diagnosed earlier.

Since ADHD impacts every part of your life, I highly encourage you to find a therapist, counselor, or social worker who understands ADHD and uses neurodiversity-affirming practices to support their clients. If you struggle with disordered eating or an eating disorder, you may also want to consider having a therapist who is trained to support you with this too. Look for a therapist who offers a discovery call so you can learn about how they support their clients and ask questions before you work with them.

Emotional dysregulation is one of the most challenging parts of my ADHD. It took me years of therapy, medication, and a lot of work on myself to get to a point where I didn't binge to regulate my emotions. Now I still eat for emotional reasons sometimes and even overeat on occasion, but I no longer binge eat to avoid feeling my feelings. **This is because I've made a crucial connection. I know now that eating until I feel ill is going to make me feel bad physically and emotionally.**

If you want to stop overeating or binge eating for emotional reasons, you have to learn how to allow yourself to feel your feelings so you can work through them.

Emotional Trigger	Eating Response
Anger, frustration	Eating as a release
Anxiety	Eating to calm the nervous system
Emotional discomfort	Eating to numb yourself from feelings
Boredom	Eating to give yourself something to do
Celebration	Eating as a reward or to connect with others
Feelings of emptiness or lack	Eating to fill unfilled spiritual or physical needs
Excitement	Eating for fun
Loneliness or feeling unloved	Eating because food feels like your friend
Mild depression	Eating carbs to increase serotonin or your "feel good" brain chemical
Procrastination	Eating to avoid starting a task
Stress or chaos	Eating to relax or get a break from a chaotic life

What Are Your Emotional Eating Triggers?

Emotions can trigger us not only to eat but also to restrict. For some emotions, it may depend on the situation. Stress is a great example of this. For some folks, stress makes them ravenous. For other people, it crushes their appetite. For others, it depends on the source of stress. Your emotional eating triggers are unique to you.

Review the list of common emotional eating triggers in the table on the left. Which trigger(s) stand out the most to you? How does this emotion impact your eating behavior? Are there certain foods you eat to deal with a certain emotion?

Interoception and Emotional Eating

As you can see, emotional dysregulation is a huge part of why ADHDers may be more prone to emotional eating. But there is another aspect of ADHD that can make this even more complicated. It's time to revisit our old friend from chapter 3: interoception.

In chapter 3, we explored how interoception differences can make it challenging to recognize and respond to body states such as hunger and fullness. These same differences can also make it hard to recognize our emotional states, which is why it's helpful for ADHDers to practice identifying emotions and the unmet needs that drive them.

Identifying the emotions you are feeling in your body can help you ground yourself in the here and now and determine your unmet needs. It can also empower you to make an intentional decision around what to do about how you are feeling. Just like learning the signs of hunger so you can eat before you feel ravenous, learning the sensations that arise with various emotions can help you become better at feeling and regulating your emotions before they feel too overwhelming.

Unmasking with Food

Masking is also referred to as camouflaging. It is the conscious or unconscious behaviors we do to appear more neurotypical. Everyone masks to some degree, but ADHDers are much more likely to mask to avoid judgment, rejection, or bullying. They may also mask to appear more successful at work or school or to make friends. While masking can serve a purpose, it is exhausting to do it all day long, and it can leave you emotionally dysregulated. Masking makes you more likely to experience depression, anxiety, and suicidal thoughts.

Part of masking is denying your sensory needs. During the day, you may not allow yourself to do things that help with your ability to focus and keep your energy up, like listening to music, using fidgets, or getting up frequently to move your body. Pushing down your intense emotions, such as frustration or excitement, is another example of masking. In the short term, denying yourself access to tools that help you focus and pushing down your feelings might help you avoid judgment and fit in, but they lead to finding unhelpful outlets, such as binge eating, to unmask when you're finally able to. Many of the tools and strategies we discuss in this chapter can serve as helpful alternatives to using food as a tool to unmask and unwind at the end of the day.

Learning How to Answer the Question "How Do I Feel?"

You need to be able to name what you're feeling before you can tame it. For many ADHDers, this can be a challenge. We tend to be more externally oriented, so we may find it difficult to tap into our internal environment. There are a couple of tools that I find useful when it comes to answering the question, "How do I feel?" One is the Feelings Thermometer.

Emotions Can Be Hunger Cues

As we discussed in chapter 3, ADHDers don't always experience a growling stomach when they are hungry. For some ADHDers, your hunger cue may be a shift in mood. If you ignore these cues, as you've learned, you may not eat enough, which can lead to the ADHD binge/restrict cycle. Diet culture would try to convince you that you did something wrong by eating because of the shift in your mood. But this is not eating purely for emotional reasons. This is learning and honoring how your hunger shows up in your body.

The Feelings Thermometer

The Feelings Thermometer not only helps you identify what you are feeling in the moment, but it also shows you what you can do to soothe this feeling.

The thermometer is divided into four colors: red, yellow, green, and blue. Each color represents a different group of emotions. If you struggle with differentiating between emotions, such as anxiety or excitement, this visual may be helpful because the feelings are grouped together. This allows you to see what strategies are suggested for similar feelings. Trying some of the strategies from feelings in the same area of the thermometer may be effective.

Red feelings are intense, explosive feelings like agitation, anger, devastation, fear, or stress. When you are feeling these emotions, you may feel as if you are actually "seeing red."

Yellow feelings can feel as if there are bees buzzing around in your head, or your stomach is filled with butterflies. These include confusion, overwhelm, embarrassment, excitement, irritation, worry, or anxiety.

Green feelings can be positive or neutral. They include feeling confident, content, focused, happy, hopeful, peaceful, or proud.

Blue feelings are like a dark, stormy day. These feelings include disappointment, rejection, boredom, sadness, or fatigue.

Just as learning what hunger feels like in your body, you may have to learn or build more awareness around what sensations show up when you are experiencing one of these emotions. Does your body temperature change? Has your breathing or heart rate changed? Do you notice any different sensations in your body? If so, what part of your body? Can you describe the sensation?

How Do You Act?

- Agitated, angry, frightened, stressed out
- Confused, embarrassed, overstimulated, avoidant
- Smiling, relaxed, laughing, engaged, paying attention
- Withdrawn, disengaged, crying, depressed

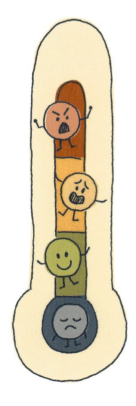

What Can You Do About It?

- Exercise, take deep breaths, take a nap, count to ten
- Take deep breaths, use positive self-talk, take a break
- Smile and practice gratitude, help someone
- Get some fresh air, listen to music, do a hobby you enjoy

Color	What You Need	Strategies
Red Feelings	To bring the temperature down (literally and figuratively)	• Vigorous movement • Taking a cold shower • Count down from 10 or 100 before you respond • Practice grounding techniques • Grab a pillow and throw it on the ground (repeat as necessary) • Listen to music that will help you process this feeling • Writing out what you are feeling
Yellow Feelings	To feel calm or more relaxed	• Meditation, breathing exercises, closing your eyes and imagining that you are in your peaceful, happy place, gentle yoga • Pause and ask for help, do a brain dump to organize your thoughts • Take a break • Practice 5 (things you can see), 4 (things you can feel), 3 (things you can hear), 2 (things you can smell), 1 (thing you can taste)
Green Feelings	To find good ways to utilize this energy	• Practice gratitude or smiling • Help others • Spend time with friends or loved ones • Move your body • Write or verbally reflect on your successes • Try something new or take action toward a goal
Blue Feelings	To feel alive or joyful	• Give or receive a hug • Listen to upbeat music • Use a scent that you have an emotional connection with • Take a nap or go to bed on time • Change up your environment • Body double, talk to a friend or family member • Dance or do something that forces you to be in your body (if that feels safe) • Do something you enjoy that requires you to be actively engaged (so not scrolling social media)

What Do I Need to Work Through This Feeling in This Moment?

Once you have identified what you are feeling, ask yourself:

"What do I need in this moment to deal with how I am feeling?"

This can help you uncover what unmet need is causing you to feel this way or making you want to turn to food to cope.

It is okay if you are not sure what you need. If you knew what you needed, it's unlikely you would be turning to food. You may need distraction, support, self-care, or the time to process that emotion directly.

The table on page 64 includes suggestions for what you might need for the red, yellow, green, and blue feelings on the Feelings Thermometer.

Asking yourself these two questions to help build awareness and promote change. What am I feeling? And what do I need in this moment to deal with this feeling? Pausing to ask yourself these questions can help you slow down and take a breath between your impulse and your action.

The more you practice asking yourself these questions, the better you will get at this. You may have to leave yourself reminders that these questions exist. You may want to have your partner or friend ask you these questions if you are emotionally dysregulated.

Building an Emotional Coping Tool Kit

Now that you've learned to identify what you're feeling and what you need to deal with it in the moment, let's build your emotional coping tool kit.

Your emotional coping tool kit is part of a larger collection of strategies to help you cope with the challenges ADHDers face. This collection should also include strategies for meeting your sensory needs (see sidebar on page 88) and for your dopamine needs, which we'll discuss in chapter 6.

It is normal and okay not to use each of your emotional coping tools daily or consistently. Some tools may be reserved for times of need and that's okay. And just because other people use a tool doesn't mean you have to.

Meeting Emotional Needs

Let's return to the Feelings Thermometer. Pick at least one feeling from each category (red, yellow, green, blue) on the thermometer. If boredom, reward, and procrastination are on your list, then I want you to save those for the next chapter when we create your Dopamenu. Usually these are signs that you are looking for stimulation.

Then follow these steps:

- Step 1: Grab a piece of paper and a pen. Set a timer for 10 minutes.
- Step 2: Pick an emotion and write: When I am feeling [insert emotion], I can do _____.
- Step 3: Under this statement, create a list of all the things that you can do to help with that emotion.

- Step 4: When the timer goes off, reset it and pick the next emotion. Repeat until you've done this for all the emotions selected.

The reason I like to start with the Feelings Thermometer for this activity is because it categorizes similar emotions together. I use similar strategies for emotions in each of these categories, so that makes sense to my brain. When I look at the Feelings Thermometer, I can pick from the menu of options to find those that will be the most helpful in the moment.

On-the-Go Self-Regulation Kit

You may want to consider creating a portable tool kit that contains a few items for self-regulation to keep in your car, purse, briefcase, or backpack. Think about how you can make accessing these tools as easy as possible so you will use them.

Maybe you have a photo folder in your phone that includes self-care things that would be helpful like the Feelings Thermometer (see page 63) or Dopamenu (see page 76), hunger/fullness cues, pictures of things you enjoy doing that you forget about.

You may even want a physical self-regulation kit. I have a little kit that I carry with me for traveling. It's a small box that contains some small fidgets, earplugs, gum, and an eye mask.

Meeting Sensory Needs

When it comes to my sensory needs, I think about tangible tools and how to set up my environment so I don't get overstimulated. One resource that has helped me in the past is *The Neurodivergent Friendly Workbook of DBT Skills* by Sonny Jane Wise. They discuss creating a sensory safe space or place where you can retreat when you feel dysregulated. For me, this is my living room.

Here are some things to consider when creating a sensory safe space:

- **Lighting:** Bright white lights can be overstimulating. I have a dimmer light switch, cool lights that allow me to adjust the color to fit my mood, and a twinkling Christmas tree (that I use all year round).

- **Sitting space:** Try to give yourself multiple seating options that fit your sensory needs. Options might include an exercise ball, swiveling barstool, or a soft floor pillow. Personally, the floor is my go-to spot to sit.

- **Tangible tools:** Think of tools that might be helpful when you feel overstimulated such as a weighted blanket, ear plugs, pictures that bring up positive memories, a sound machine, fuzzy socks, or a yoga mat.

What Do I Do If I Want to Emotionally Eat?

If you choose to emotionally eat, then do so without judgment or shame. I find it helpful to label it and to make a moment out of it if I can. While writing this book, my family dog of seventeen years passed away. I was heartbroken. I wanted something to bring me some joy, so while grocery shopping, I bought a big cookie at the register. Later that day, I said out loud to myself, "I am going to eat as much of this cookie as I want because I am feeling sad." I sat on my couch with my dogs, ate my cookie, and cried. I knew the cookie wouldn't fix how I was feeling. But I needed a short break from feeling sad, and the cookie met that need.

Create a Boundary to Curb Emotional Eating

If you are not physically or mentally restricting but find that you are opting for food in place of other coping strategies, then you may want to explore creating a boundary with yourself. The purpose of this boundary is to help create enough space to utilize your other coping tools.

Maybe this boundary is bringing enough of the snacks that you typically eat during the day to stay regulated and not feel deprived at work. The key piece here would be allowing yourself to eat them without judgment or guilt.

Maybe you have a boundary that you put food in a bowl or on a plate and sit down to eat it more intentionally. This may work for some, but for others this may just turn into a food rule. I would truly only make a boundary like this if you know that you are actively picking food in place of other coping tools and not because you feel this will give you self-control with food.

Think of your boundaries as temporarily removing the emotional eating trigger to allow you to choose the opposite action for once. If you really want that food, you can honor that feeling and eat it.

Urge Surfing

Urge surfing is acknowledging that you have an urge (for example, to emotionally eat or binge eat) and hitting the pause button on acting on it. You can't always prevent an urge, but you can choose how you respond to it. Urge surfing means that you are practicing delaying or putting space between the urge and the action. It helps your brain learn that you can tolerate this feeling.

When using this strategy, you may want to determine in advance the minimum amount of time you will ride the urge wave. It could be as short as 60 seconds. You may also want to make a list of activities you can do while you are riding the wave to help you stay busy or feel calm. Refer to your emotional coping tool kit to help with this.

Steps to Urge Surfing

1. **Identify the urge** by saying to yourself: "I am feeling the urge to binge eat because [insert binge trigger]. Just because I am feeling this urge doesn't mean that I am required to respond to it."
2. **Decide how long** you will surf the urge wave. It may be helpful to determine this in advance. It could be as short as 60 seconds.
3. **Pick** an activity to do or find somewhere comfortable to sit down.
4. **Set a timer** for that amount of time.
5. When it goes off can you go for another 60 seconds? **Repeat as many times** as you can or until the urge passes.
6. After you ride the wave, **give yourself praise** for trying it instead of immediately giving in to the urge.
7. **Reflect with curiosity instead of judgment:** What went well? What didn't go so well? What would you do differently in the future?

Make It a Habit to Check in With Yourself to See How You're Feeling

Learning to pause and check in with yourself is a practice. It will take time, patience, and repetition to develop. It may not come naturally to you, but that doesn't mean it's not something worth doing. Checking in with yourself to see how you are feeling and what you need not only helps with regulating your emotions, but it also helps with meeting other bodily needs. If you never make space to do this, life will become chaotic and you will get into the ADHD burnout cycle—starting a task, being interrupted by ADHD traits, which then leads to stress and turning to unhelpful coping tools, like avoidance, procrastination, and self-medicating, until you feel so stuck that you quit or withdraw.

As I mentioned in chapter 4, it can be helpful to set an alarm for self check-in during the day and label it "What do I need?"

You may want to add the question "What am I feeling?" to this alarm. I recommend setting an alarm during a stretch(es) of time where you may need to be reminded to check in wit=h yourself or maybe after something that may be emotionally draining for you.

Create a Self-Care Checklist

When I am really busy or stressed, I don't always remember to make time to check in with myself or do things that will help me function my best and stay regulated, such as eating lunch. So, I created a checklist of what I would *ideally* like to get done during my morning, midday, and afternoon routines to help me automate my check-in. This way I don't have to think about the basic tasks I need to do throughout the day to stay regulated. After waking up, it's a lot easier for me to transition

Remember F.U.N.

This acronym might help you remember, "What am I **F**eeling? What is my **U**nmet **N**eed?" The better you get at meeting your basic needs regularly, the more space you will have in your life for fun. See if you can reframe the practice of identifying a feeling and unmet need as FUN.

Sample Check-in Checklist:

AM

- ☐ Take dogs outside
- ☐ Feed dogs
- ☐ Walk Lola
- ☐ Meditate
- ☐ Cook
- ☐ Eat breakfast
- ☐ Review calendar
- ☐ Make to-do list

Mid-day

- ☐ Take dogs outside
- ☐ Make lunch (if needed)
- ☐ Eat lunch
- ☐ Dopamine snack

PM

- ☐ Take dogs outside
- ☐ Journal
- ☐ Dopamine snack
- ☐ Cook
- ☐ Eat dinner
- ☐ Review to-do list
- ☐ Closing duties

into my morning routine or from work to my midday break when I have some predetermined activities that I know I'll do to meet my basic needs.

Let me be clear—I don't do everything on this list every day because I know that I am consistently inconsistent and sometimes I don't have enough time. When I don't, I try my best to do at least one thing because I know that when I don't check in with myself, I'll feel more dysregulated, which requires me to spend more time and energy to get myself regulated again.

Make Time for Reflection

I guarantee that you have two minutes somewhere in your day when you can reflect or check in with yourself. Reflection can take many forms such as free journaling, taking voice notes using your phone, or adding notes to a daily self-reflection journal with prompts. You can verbally reflect with a friend, partner, or loved one at the end of the day or reflect by drawing or painting or playing an instrument. Maybe how you reflect changes based on what you feel like doing.

If you forget, don't beat yourself up. Think about what you can do differently tomorrow or that day to make time for it. Maybe it's moving your journal somewhere where you will see it. Maybe it's asking your partner to give you two minutes to journal before you start watching TV at night.

The more you practice checking in with yourself, the more naturally it will come to you. When you feel something in your body, stop and ask yourself, "What am I feeling? What do I need in this moment?"

Externalizing the Check-In

This strategy will require you to ask a partner or friend for help checking in with yourself. Explain that you are working on developing the habit of asking yourself the two questions so you can get better at meeting your needs and regulating your emotions but that you sometimes forget. Ask them to remind you to take a deep breath and prompt you to ask the two questions on days when they notice you are "off." Or ask them to cue you in whatever way you find helpful.

Remember that the goal is not to rely on them to check in with you but to cue you until it becomes part of your natural routine. For me, 90 percent of the time I simply need to be reminded to eat, hydrate, get fresh air, or foster social connection.

Emotional hunger is a huge, complicated topic for ADHDers, and learning how to manage it is a key part of healing your relationship with food. In the next chapter, we'll discuss a topic that's closely related: brain hunger, or eating for stimulation.

CHAPTER 6

ADHD: The Food and Dopamine Connection

Dopamine is our "feel good" neurotransmitter or brain chemical messenger. It helps with motivation, concentration, and regulating our emotions. It allows you to feel pleasure when you listen to music, pet a dog, exercise, or eat your favorite food. Dopamine is involved in so many mental and physical functions that regulating this brain chemical is important for everyone's overall health. But I would argue that ADHDers need even more attention to support our low dopamine brains.

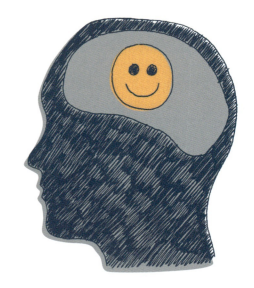

In ADHD brains, dopamine levels and functioning are different. Neurotypical brains get dopamine during a task, in anticipation of completing it and for achieving a positive outcome. But ADHDers get it from things we find interesting or enjoyable. So completing boring tasks feels less rewarding. Additionally, any dopamine you do get does not last as long as it does for someone who does not have ADHD. This leads to struggles with motivation, procrastination, and task avoidance. Lastly, in the past decade we have started to study the connection between estrogen and ADHD and discovered that when estrogen levels drop, such as in the luteal phase of the menstrual cycle or in menopause, dopamine levels also appear to drop. This impacts how ADHD presents in women and folks assigned female at birth.

Such alterations in dopamine levels and pathways play a role in ADHD and in substance use disorders and eating disorders. So, it's not surprising that ADHDers are at a significantly higher risk of developing both. This is why it is critical for ADHDers to learn how to support their brain's dopamine levels.

In this chapter, we are going to explore the dopamine-food connection, what eating for stimulation looks like, the pros and cons of using food for stimulation, and how to build a tool kit to address your need for stimulation.

The Dopamine-Food Connection

Everyone experiences dopamine after eating food. Throughout history, humans have needed to experience feelings of pleasure or feel rewarded for eating food to ensure they would seek it out when there wasn't enough to stay alive. There is still A LOT of research that needs to be done to understand individual variations in dopamine production in response to food. Based on the research currently available, here are some things we do know.

When you see, smell, and taste food, it increases your dopamine levels. Our desire to eat a particular food and our hunger levels also appear to influence how much dopamine is produced in response to eating a food. This means that the hungrier you are or the more you enjoy a food, the more dopamine your body releases. So when you are ravenous and instinctually reach for something you really love like simple carbs, sweets, or snack food, it's partly because you're getting a lot more dopamine from those foods in that moment.

For most folks, food is a pretty low-effort, accessible, and enjoyable source of dopamine. This can lead ADHDers to rely too much on food to get dopamine. Food is often used alongside other tasks such as studying, watching TV, or working to increase stimulation and help you stay focused. The downside of this is that you might get so focused on that task that you are unable to regulate how much you're eating or connect with how full you feel.

Dopamine and Eating Disorders

The development of eating disorders is complex and multifactorial, but dopamine is a big part of why ADHDers are more likely to struggle with binge eating disorder (BED) and bulimia nervosa. Researchers have identified alterations to dopamine pathways in the brain that contribute to BED and bulimia nervosa. But more research is needed to fully understand

Stimming

ADHD brains are constantly seeking ways to regulate their dopamine levels. We often fluctuate between under stimulation and overstimulation. One way that ADHDers regulate dopamine levels is by stimming. Stimming is repetitive physical movements or sounds that help soothe, regulate sensory input, and release energy. For ADHDers, fidgeting has been shown to help with focusing to complete tasks that are uninteresting or not stimulating enough to your brain. It can also be a way to soothe feelings of anxiety, stress, or nervousness.

Food is a great example of a tool for stimulation that can be helpful, but if it leads to overeating or binge eating, it can be harmful. Most of the time, though, stimming behaviors are harmless.

these alterations. As an ADHDer who's binged as well as binged and purged, I always felt as if there was a part of my experience that was missing from conversations about eating disorders. That missing piece was that what I really needed was to get my brain dopamine, and I was using these behaviors to do it.

I remember going on a vacation where I didn't take my meds, didn't restrict or binge, and generally had a great time. When I got home, I binged and purged. This didn't make sense to me. Years later, I learned that this is a common way to manage the dopamine crash after an activity that gave you a lot of dopamine.

Pros and Cons of Eating for Stimulation

Yes, eating food is an easy and accessible way to get dopamine. It's a form of self-medication that can help you regulate your attention, mood, and energy levels—all good things! It also serves as a reminder that some of life's simplest pleasures can be a source of dopamine.

On the other hand, eating for stimulation can lead to overeating and binge eating, which don't make you feel good. Binge eating can negatively impact your health long-term. It can increase your risk for type 2 diabetes, high blood pressure, high cholesterol, heart disease, gallbladder disease, and some cancers. ADHDers tend to seek out hyperpalatable foods for stimulation. These foods are usually more energy- or calorie-dense. Eating more energy than what your body needs can also lead to weight gain. This is one possible reason why people who have ADHD are more likely to live in larger bodies.

It's not helpful or realistic to suggest that ADHDers should never eat for stimulation. That would be like telling a kid with ADHD that they cannot fidget in class. Many ADHDers feel shame around eating for stimulation, especially if it leads to binge eating. But you're not a bad person or a failure if you eat for emotional reasons or for stimulation. Trying to avoid eating for stimulation is a form of restriction.

The goal is not to eliminate eating for stimulation. The goal is to add other sources of stimulation to your life so that food is not the only source. And if you choose to eat for stimulation, you are able to do so without guilt. Just like eating for emotional reasons, eating for stimulation can serve a purpose.

ADHD Medication & Dopamine

There are a variety of medications used in ADHD management. These include stimulants, nonstimulants, and antidepressants.

Stimulants, specifically amphetamines, are the first-line treatment for managing ADHD in adults. These medications help increase levels of dopamine and norepinephrine in the brain. In theory, nonstimulants also increase the concentrations of these neurotransmitters in the prefrontal cortex of the brain. But nonstimulants can take between four and eight weeks to reach their maximum benefits. With stimulants you will notice their effect within an hour.

Decreased appetite is a common side effect on ADHD meds. As previously discussed, dopamine plays a role in regulating food intake. When your brain gets enough dopamine from meds, it signals to your stomach that you are full—even if you haven't eaten. Alternatively, having enough dopamine means that you can get so focused that you forget to eat.

Friendly reminder—regulating appetite is not the purpose of these medications, and using stimulants to restrict your food intake is a sign of disordered eating or a potential eating disorder.

How Do I Know If I Am Physically Hungry or Seeking Stimulation?

Knowing why you want to eat can help you make more intentional choices. Seeking stimulation from food may feel like boredom eating, eating to procrastinate, or eating as a reward. Stimulation eating can also result from needing to do something with your hands or mouth. You might seek out a very specific taste or texture to satisfy your need for stimulation.

As we suggested in the previous chapter, get into the habit of checking in with yourself. Be curious. If you're experiencing any physical signs of hunger, give yourself permission to honor your hunger. If you don't feel any signs of hunger, when was the last time you ate? If it's been three or more hours since you last ate, it might be time to eat something. If it hasn't been three or more hours, are you feeling bored, like you need to do something with your hands or mouth, or like your brain is trying to scratch an itch? If yes, this is likely your brain telling you it needs stimulation. Would mindfully eating help? Or would something else feel more helpful in this moment?

It's totally okay if you choose to eat for stimulation if that feels helpful. If it doesn't, try to use other tools for the stimulation you seek. (We'll talk more about this later.) This is especially true if you know mindlessly eating for stimulation will lead to you overeating or binge eating. One of the most common ways I see food being used for stimulation in a way that leads to overeating or bingeing is eating while watching TV, scrolling social media, etc. This is because doing those things alone is often not stimulating enough for ADHD brains. I keep fidgets, a coloring book, a balance board, and a cross stitch in my living room so I can do other things while I watch TV besides doomscroll or eat when I'm not actually hungry.

How Restriction and Inconsistent Eating Patterns Affects Dopamine

Restricting food increases the reward value or the dopamine you are getting from those foods. The foods you crave are often the foods you have the most physical or mental restrictions around. If you are restricting foods, dieting, or have extensive food rules, you are increasing the reward value of these foods by avoiding them. Our brains get more dopamine from things that are off-limits, which may explain part of why we might get into harmful behaviors.

I have found, when you make peace with food and explore other tools for stimulation, food doesn't give you the same dopamine hit it does when you try to make it off-limits.

As I've said, if you are not eating enough during the day, going four or more hours without eating, or coming out of a chronic period of restriction/dieting, then it is very likely that you are actually physically hungry instead of just needing dopamine.

Honor Your Brain Hunger

Interoception differences can also make it difficult to know if what we're feeling is physical hunger or brain hunger (needing stimulation). One reason I think it's important to normalize all forms of hunger is that so many ADHDers shame themselves for honoring brain hunger, but this is a valid reason to eat!

Eating for stimulation may also be paired with eating for emotional regulation (including in response to stress, which is more about serotonin than dopamine). ADHD meds help regulate emotions, so when they wear off, you might turn to food to deal with emotions you may have not properly dealt with during the day. This can create a perfect storm for binge eating; you may be undereating, experiencing stress from work, and looking for stimulation.

What you eat and when you eat also influence dopamine signaling. This is why it is so important to work toward developing a more regular eating pattern. Refer to chapter 4 to find an eating pattern that will help set you on the path to eating regularly.

How Do You Use Food for Stimulation?

If you want to decrease how much you rely on food for stimulation, the first step is to understand when and why you use food in this way. The following questions will help you identify when you may turn to food for dopamine.

- Are there certain activities or tasks that prompt you to feel as if you need food to help you focus? Examples might include studying, driving, filling out spreadsheets, etc.
- What tastes and textures make your brain happy? Tastes include sweet, sour, or spicy, while textures might be crunchy, chewy, or gummy.
- Are you more likely to eat for stimulation during certain times of the day, such as the evening, or at particular times during the year, such as studying for finals in college?
- Does where you are at in your menstrual cycle impact how much you use food for stimulation?

During these times, easy, quick sources of dopamine, like food, might not be meeting your needs in the ways that you would like. Later in the chapter you'll learn new ways to stimulate a dopamine response.

Maximize Eating for Stimulation When You Do

If you are going to eat for stimulation, try to make the most of the experience so you can maximize the dopamine you are getting from food. *Slow down* and focus on the sensory qualities of the food. Do you notice the fudgy texture and rich chocolate flavor of the brownie you're eating while you type an email? Or do you finish the brownie only to realize you have no recollection of eating it so you sneak back to the break room for more?

It may sound cheesy, but romanticizing or making a moment out of eating for stimulation can help limit distractions so you're able to notice more of the sensory aspects of the food. So maybe instead of eating the brownie while you write an email, you take a five-minute break to step outside for fresh air and eat it at a picnic table. Pay attention to the aroma, taste, and texture of the food. Being more mindful of how you feel when you're eating provides more satisfaction. This makes it easier to stop when you're full.

Eating for Stimulation at Work

Work is often one of the most challenging environments when it comes to eating for stimulation. That's because it requires more stimulation to accomplish, but you don't always have time to meet this need. If you work in a stressful, high-demand job, then you might find you eat for stimulation and emotional dysregulation. Do you:

- **Graze throughout the day?** When you do this, you'll never be satiated. You may eat like this during the day because your meds zap your appetite, so you don't eat enough food and feel ravenous when they wear off at night. Or you eat this way because you are self-medicating with food and don't pause for meals.
- **Allow yourself to eat for stimulation, but hold on to guilty thoughts or beat yourself up for it?** You approach it from an all-or-nothing mindset. When you "give in" by having just one cookie, piece of candy, chip, etc., then you tell yourself, "Screw it, I might as well just keep eating because I've blown it or messed it up."
- **Eat while doing one or more other things?** You eat fast, especially if you are ashamed about it, and don't even allow yourself a moment to enjoy it.

If you do any of the things listed above, you'll benefit from finding other tools for stimulation at work. You will also have to accept that sometimes you'll still eat for stimulation, especially if your job or job setting limits what tools you have access to.

Other Tools to Stimulate Dopamine

I don't like referring to sources of dopamine as "good vs. bad" or "healthy vs. unhealthy" for the same reasons I don't like to use these labels with food—it creates shame and judgment, which do not help with behavior change. Instead, **I like to think of dopamine sources as helpful, less helpful, or unhelpful.** This helps you explore what you can do for stimulation from a place of curiosity. If you think that nothing but food will give you dopamine, then nothing will, so I encourage you to keep an open, curious mind when it comes to seeking other tools.

Getting your ADHD brain dopamine is part of self-care for ADHDers. It is a basic need for us. We need it to function properly. Medication can be an incredible tool for this reason. But if you don't make time to get dopamine from other sources, then keeping your ADHD managed will be challenging. Meds will not fix everything. Even if meds give you the dopamine you need to function optimally, adding other stimulating activities will extend the battery life.

Give yourself permission to do things that allow you to experience pleasure and enjoyment on a daily basis. These can be big activities, like going to a concert, or smaller activities, like enjoying your favorite fizzy water. You are allowed to do things that make you feel good and that are important to you. Doing so will help you live a more fulfilling life.

In the next section we will learn how to build a "menu" of options for when you need to serve up some dopamine. This is called a "Dopamenu."

Building Your Dopamenu

In chapter 5, we talked about building an emotional coping tool kit. This section is about building a similar tool kit for stimulation. This tool kit will not only include tangible tools, like fidget toys or crochet yarn, but it will also include less tangible tools, like dancing or spending time outside. The "Dopamenu" is a visual representation of this tool kit. It was created by Eric Tivers of *ADHD reWired* and Jessica McCabe of *How to ADHD*.

One frustrating aspect of ADHD is forgetting what tools and strategies you have in the moment. This can lead to defaulting to less helpful tools and strategies, like eating or doomscrolling or getting stuck in ADHD paralysis. The Dopamenu helps avoid this.

Creating and using a Dopamenu can help you find motivation, start, continue, or stop a task and help you unwind from overstimulation. For me, understanding that my brain is constantly seeking dopamine has really helped me better understand myself and my behaviors. When you are meeting your dopamine needs, you will have more capacity to do other tasks in your life and take better care of yourself. It can help you build trust in your innate wisdom to know what you want or need.

Since ADHDers crave novelty, you will need to update your Dopamenu regularly with new activities. But first, let's discuss what a Dopamenu actually looks like and how to build one.

What Is a Dopamenu?

Just as you use a menu at a restaurant to select what you want to eat, you can use your Dopamenu to select what activity will help you get dopamine in that moment. The six sections of the Dopamenu I use are starters, sides, mains, specials, desserts, and late-night snacks. Each section represents a different type of activity that helps create dopamine in your brain.

Your Dopamenu will be unique to you and your interests. What one person might consider an appetizer, another person might think of as dessert. (Keep in mind that food can be a part of your Dopamenu and it can fit into multiple categories.) Let's take a look at each category in turn, with examples.

Starters

Think of your starters as a quick burst of dopamine. They do not require a lot of time, money, or effort. Starters can make it easier to initiate a task, be it a small reward for completing a task, or a fun short break.

Examples:

- The ritual of making a cup of coffee or tea
- Shaking it (your body) out
- 10-minute guided meditation
- Listen or dance to an upbeat song
- Call a friend
- Race the clock to see if you can complete a certain activity within a certain amount of time you set on a timer
- Changing environments
- Cheering for yourself when you complete a boring task
- Lighting a candle when you start a task

Sides

A side is anything that makes it easier for you to do another task. They can help make a task more fun or interesting or even more motivating so that you actually get it done. Sides should be tools that engage one of your other senses that you are not using to do a task.

Examples:

- Fidgets (squishy ball, spinner, pop-it toy, etc.)
- Gum
- Chewelry or chewable jewelry
- Knitting or crochet
- Doing a puzzle
- Crunchy snacks (carrots, nuts, apples, salt and vinegar chips)
- Listening to music, a podcast, or an audiobook
- Body doubling (see page 125)
- Talking on the phone or FaceTiming
- Using colored PaperMate InkJoy pens
- Carbonated drinks such as Olipop or carbonated water
- Using a balance board instead of sitting
- Using a walking pad or desk bike at work

Mains

Mains are activities that take more time and energy than an appetizer but provide you with more dopamine. These are activities that you enjoy and benefit from doing. Your special interests would fall into this category. Mains may be things you do that really help with managing your ADHD.

Examples:

- Going for a walk with your dog.
- Going for a run or doing High Intensity Interval Training (HIIT)
- Cooking a meal or baking cookies
- Spending quality time with friends, family members, or a partner
- Crafting or painting
- Completing a project
- Learning about your current hyperfixation/special interest
- Learning a new skill or hobby
- Longer meditation or somatic dance class
- Sex
- Playing a sport with a rec team
- Going to bed on time
- Getting sunlight or enjoying a green space

Specials

As the name implies, these are special activities that you may not be able to do on a regular basis because they require more time, money, and effort than the other categories. These might be things that you easily forget you enjoy because you don't get to do them as regularly. You may be able to use your specials more often if you have more disposable income.

Examples:

- Dinner and drinks at a nice restaurant
- Weekend trip
- Manicure/pedicure
- Massage or facial
- Going to see a movie
- Going to a music festival or concert
- Going to a sporting event
- Buying yourself a bouquet of flowers or a plant

Desserts

Like true desserts, these are activities that can be easy to overdo and may not be as fulfilling. They give you little bursts of dopamine, and that makes you want to come back for more. It's pretty unrealistic to say you are never going to eat dessert for the rest of your life, however these activities may be things that you want to limit or that you may need specific boundaries around. If you forget that certain activities don't fulfill you as much until after you do them, then hopefully this can help you choose better in the moment.

Examples:

- Sweets, snacky foods
- Sugar sweetened beverages
- Caffeine
- Doomscrolling social media
- Impulse or online shopping
- Picking fights or starting arguments when bored
- Body focused repetitive behaviors (skin picking or hair pulling)
- Excessive exercise
- Binge watching TV

Late-Night Snacks

I stumbled upon this section when looking at sample Dopamenus online. Late-night snacks are activities and tools that can help you wind down or help when you are overstimulated. Often, I see folks looking for stimulation when really their brain is looking for a way to deal with too much stimulation.

This happens a lot in the evening. Instead of trying to wind down their brain from all the stimulation it got all day, they keep looking for more ways to get dopamine and stay awake. Your late-night snacks might be things that help you end your day without turning to activities in your desserts category, like binge eating or bingeing your favorite show and staying up until 2:00 am. It's okay to slow down a little. These things may help manage the crash from being overstimulated.

Examples:

- Chill playlist
- Sleep aids:
  - Lavender pillow mist or essential oil
  - Dim lights, eye mask, or ear plugs
  - White noise machine
  - Weighted blanket or pillow
- Squishmallow
- Skincare routine
- Cuddling with a pet or loved one
- Journaling
- Stretching
- Getting things ready for tomorrow (laying out clothes, making breakfast or lunch, tidying living space, etc.) so your future self is set up for success
- Laying down and closing your eyes for 15 minutes (midday sensory break)
- Mood lighting or fairy lights
- Changing into soft or sensory friendly clothes after work
- Alone time after events involving masking

How Do I Make My Dopamenu?

If you're creating a Dopamenu for the first time, I recommend following three simple steps.

Step One: Brainstorm Ways to Stimulate Dopamine

First, google Dopamenu to get an idea of how you want yours to look. Next, set a timer for 20 to 30 minutes. Get out a piece of paper and draw a vertical line down the middle of the page. On the left side, write out all the possible activities that you could put on your Dopamenu. These are activities that you find exciting, fun, and make you feel alive.

Moira Maybin, an ADHD podcaster, coach, and educator, recommends writing out things that provide some of the acronym **P.I.N.C.H.,** which stands for **P**lay; **I**nterest; **N**ovelty; **C**ompetition, **C**ollaboration & **C**onnection; or **H**urry up (or create sense of urgency). If you can, do this activity with another ADHDer in your life so you can bounce ideas off each other and make it a fun experience. If you struggle with coming up with things you enjoy, take some time to get curious and reflect on it for a bit. There is no judgment about what you find enjoyable. Some of these activities may be typically thought of as something that is for kids, but you are allowed to play and make your inner child happy.

Step Two: Review Your List and Narrow It Down

Once you've created your master list of stimulating activities, set another timer for 30 to 40 minutes. On the right side of the page, write all the activities that you can feasibly do right now. For example, if it's summer, don't write skiing on the right side of the page because that's not a feasible activity for you right now.

Step Three: Categorize and Create Your Dopamenu

Next, review each category of the Dopamenu and sort your activities into each one.

Remember, your Dopamenu is a living document, so you can always add tools to or remove them from this menu. Don't stress if you can't fill it out all at once.

Once you've got the basic structure and content down, it's time for the fun part. Make your Dopamenu visually appealing and an expression of who you are. Consider using icons alone or with text. For example, you could draw a stick figure holding a yoga pose or use emojis. Once it's complete, keep your Dopamenu in a place that's visible, such as on your refrigerator, the door of your pantry, the lock screen on your phone, or at your desk.

How Do I Make Using My Dopamenu a Practice?

First, give yourself permission and create time and space to be able to do things on your Dopamenu. Keep it visible and in multiple places so you remember it exists. Keep it in your kitchen to remind you of other things you can do when you are looking for stimulation and not actually hungry. You may want to have a reminder or alarm on your phone or calendar to look at your Dopamenu.

For activities you want to do more of, think about how you can lower the roadblocks and barriers to them. I leave fidget toys on my coffee table as a visual cue instead of wandering to the pantry when I am not hungry. Maybe you'll want to keep food in the pantry instead of on the counter. You know that it is available and an option, but there are more barriers to it.

You can also add more roadblocks and barriers to decrease less helpful activities in other areas of your life. I have my apps that shut off my phone to help me go to bed earlier and prevent doomscrolling. While I can and do hit the "remind me in 15 minutes button, it at least helps me be more aware of how long I am on my phone not doing anything.

Sometimes it can be hard to start and stop some activities. Restricting yourself from enjoyable activities can lead to wanting to rebel or binge on things you enjoy. Food may be one of the things you restrict, or it might be what you turn to because you don't make space for other activities. Please give yourself permission to do things on this list regularly without guilt or shame.

Think of dopamine like a battery. Making time to do things that provide you with enjoyment and make you feel fulfilled will help keep your battery charged. Your battery will drain more quickly if you do not make time for these things in your life, and when your battery runs out of juice, it will likely take a lot more effort and time to get your battery recharged. This is why the ADHD burnout cycle can be hard to escape from.

Just like it's a lot easier to stop eating a food when you don't deprive yourself of it and your body knows it will be available later, it's a lot easier to stop these activities when you know you can do them again.

Reframe being bored, looking for a reward, or procrastinating as a sign that your brain is looking for dopamine, and refer to your Dopamenu to decide what you can do to get your ADHD brain the dopamine it is seeking.

Carve Out Time Every Day for Dopamine Snacks

If you are bingeing at night on food, TV, social media, alcohol, etc., then you may not be making enough time for enjoyment or pleasure in your day without guilt. Or perhaps, the ways that you are getting dopamine during the day just aren't enough or fulfilling.

This is similar to the ADHD binge/restrict cycle. Just as you need to eat enough and regularly to break this cycle, you have to regularly add enjoyment during your day or you will stay up late trying to fit it in. This is often referred to as revenge bedtime procrastination.

For this reason, I regularly carve out time in my day for what I call dopamine snacks. I use my Dopamenu to decide what dopamine snack I want to do when that time comes. This allows me to be intentional about adding helpful ways to get dopamine throughout the day. Seeing a dopamine snack on my midday checklist is something that I look forward to. Seeing it motivates me to get the other things done so that I can do my dopamine snack. You can use these snacks to transition from one task to another or use them to give yourself a break from work that is more productive than doomscrolling on your phone.

Some of my dopamine snacks include a literal snack—usually something with a crunch. If you feel as if you don't have enough time in your day to do this, then maybe start by adding some starters to your day instead of a main or special that takes up more time.

Managing dopamine levels is crucial for managing your ADHD and eating behaviors. Certainly, food can be one of your tools for stimulation, but as you've seen, it's important to create a tool kit so that you have other options to choose from as you need them. The Dopamenu is an excellent tool to help you visualize and categorize your sources of stimulation.

Now that you've learned about how to support your ADHD brain's dopamine needs, let's talk about gentle nutrition for ADHD, or what foods can support your ADHD brain.

CHAPTER 7

Gentle Nutrition for ADHD and Why It Matters

Gentle nutrition is the last principle of Intuitive Eating. This was done by design to prevent it from morphing into another unsustainable diet with a bunch of rules to follow. Gentle nutrition is about pairing your inner wisdom about how foods make you feel with general nutrition guidelines to achieve healthful eating patterns.

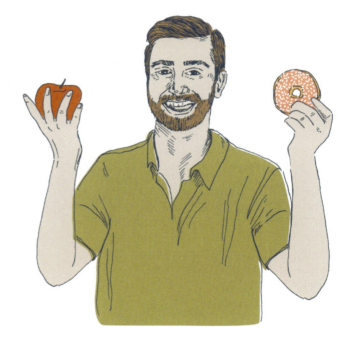

If you have a terrible relationship with food and chaotic eating patterns, then it's important to address these issues first, before trying to implement the recommendations in this chapter.

For so many ADHDers, it's not that they don't know the importance of eating nutritious food. It's that the features of ADHD, such as executive dysfunction, the need for dopamine, lack of appetite due to meds, and sensory sensitivities become HUGE barriers to actually eating well. Plus, most nutrition advice is not catered to ADHDers. I hope this chapter offers clarity and helps remove some of those barriers.

Remember, IE is not about perfect eating—that doesn't exist. When you try to make changes to your eating patterns or add more nutrient-dense foods to your diet, **focus on progress, not perfection.** This means focusing on small actions every day that can help you work toward your goal. When I work with clients, I don't expect them to completely change their diet overnight. I wouldn't expect you to either. If you've tried this before, you know it often doesn't end the way you want it to.

Diets and ADHD

Before we discuss what gentle nutrition is, let's talk about what it isn't: a diet. You may be wondering if diet can cause ADHD. The short answer is no. Research has consistently demonstrated that diet does not cause ADHD.

Inattention and hyperactivity are associated with "unhealthy eating habits" such as higher added sugar and saturated fat intake, no matter your age, sex, or socioeconomic status. However, you did not get ADHD because you ate "too much" sugar, food dyes, or processed foods. This is a common myth that needs to be debunked. If you ate a lot of sugar as a kid or even as an adult, it was to stimulate your ADHD brain. It makes sense that you would turn to easily accessible and pleasurable sources of dopamine for stimulation and emotional regulation if unmanaged ADHD was making your life feel chaotic and miserable. (We discuss some better ways of achieving this in chapters 5 and 6.)

Nutrition is also not considered a primary treatment strategy for ADHD. A review of nutrition in the management of ADHD published in 2023 found that the current "evidence from recent research does not allow any recommendations regarding the use of micronutrients or probiotics in the management of ADHD."

Historically, ADHD research, especially in regard to nutrition, has focused on kids. These studies show that diet is nowhere near as effective as medication and only provides some benefits to a subset of kids with ADHD. Even if research showed diets helped kids with ADHD, it's hard to say if those benefits would be seen in adults, because our brains are fully developed. Despite some newer studies indicating that diet may help, more studies are needed with larger sample sizes, longer duration, and stronger designs.

The 3 Guiding Principles of Nutrition

Intuitive Eating incorporates three guiding principles in nutrition: variety, moderation, and balance.

1. Variety: Different foods contain different nutrients. Aim to eat at least one food from each of the food groups. Then work toward expanding to include more foods within all the food groups.

2. Moderation: This means avoiding the extremes of not eating enough and eating too much of any given food. Moderation in IE is not elimination or trying to eat as little as possible. When you've made peace with food, you will be able to eat all foods in moderation.

3. Balance: A meal, day, or week of eating isn't going to make or break your health. It's more important to zoom out and look at your overall eating patterns. Both balance and moderation can help you challenge black and white thinking around food.

Common "Recommended" Diets for ADHD and What the Research Says

At the time this book was written, there were no peer-reviewed studies on using dietary interventions to manage ADHD in adults (there is one study currently underway). In this section, I am going to share some diets that have been studied for ADHD, what the research shows, and what to consider before starting these often very restrictive diets. Please note my discussion of these diets are not an endorsement of them.

Feingold Diet

The Feingold Diet is an elimination diet developed in the 1970s by Dr. Benjamin Feingold. This diet recommends you remove artificial flavorings, artificial sweeteners, salicylates, certain preservatives, and food dyes from your diet. This is where the myth that ADHD is caused by food dyes comes from.

The Feingold Diet has not been shown to be effective. Research shows there is a subset of children with and without ADHD that appear to respond poorly to food dyes. Removing food dyes may *insignificantly* improve ADHD traits, and researchers consider it of mild relevance.

The implementation of this diet is extremely challenging even in a research setting. If you notice removing certain foods improve your symptoms, you can cut them out. However, eliminating food dyes and additives requires a lot of extra work in the form of reading labels, spending more time and energy making foods from scratch, and spending more money, as the alternatives free of these additives tend to be more expensive. I do try to limit these things in my own diet because I tend to feel better, but I'm not overly strict.

The Few Foods Diet

Out of all of the elimination diets studied, the Few Foods Diet shows the most promise as a potential option for *kids who are too young or not a candidate for ADHD medication*. This diet is extremely restrictive during the elimination phase (you're only allowed to eat lamb/venison, quinoa/rice, pear, and veggies), and it can take up to one year to complete the reintroduction phase to figure out what foods increase your ADHD traits. That's a big ask for folks who are consistently inconsistent and struggle with impulsivity. If you've spent months trying to figure out the right meds, imagine a year on an extremely restrictive diet.

This diet may be easier for kids to follow because they have less autonomy over their food choices and are not involved in the purchasing or preparation of food. But I also think overly restrictive diets regardless of age can trigger unnecessary food fears and disordered eating in a population more prone to eating disorders in the first place. Such a diet may also increase the risk for nutrient deficiencies. In my opinion, this is a bad trade-off.

Studies on this diet also have a huge risk for observer bias, as the parents know what diet their kid is on and are the ones reporting changes in the child's behavior. Often, these are parents motivated to use more natural strategies and want their child to make improvements.

Most ADHDers I know and work with can't stick to a traditional diet for more than a few months. I'm not sure how ADHD adults would be able to do this diet without living in an isolated bubble. In fact, researchers studying this diet say that while it does show promise, it's not ready to be used outside of the research setting.

Gluten-Free Diet

Unless you have Celiac disease or non-Celiac gluten sensitivity, you do not need to eliminate gluten. The only way to determine if you are sensitive to gluten is to remove it from your diet for at least two weeks to see if you notice a difference in how you feel (you cannot test for gluten sensitivity).

If you feel better not eating gluten without these diagnoses, don't eat it. There is no strong evidence to support removing gluten from the diet to help with ADHD symptoms *unless* you have these gastrointestinal (GI) conditions. This also applies to dairy and soy—you do not need to eliminate foods containing dairy or soy unless you have an allergy or intolerance.

Ketogenic Diet

Did you know the ketogenic diet was created as a treatment for epilepsy in children? A true ketogenic diet is high in fat (about 90 percent of daily calories), moderate in protein, and low in carbohydrates (under 50 grams per day). There is some research to show it may help with Alzheimer's and Parkinson's disease, but this diet has not been studied in humans with ADHD yet.

Many people who claim to eat "keto" are doing a modified version that is basically like the Atkins diet. This version of keto is low-carb, but it's high-protein and moderate fat intake. A low-carb diet has also not been studied for ADHD yet.

Regardless, severely restricting your body's primary energy source, carbohydrates, makes it very challenging to adhere to these diets long-term. It's not sustainable and will likely do more harm than good. Weight cycling, or losing and regaining weight, can be harmful and usually happens when folks yo-yo on and off diets.

Probiotics and ADHD

This is a fascinating emerging area of research. Gut health is certainly important for our overall health but we still need a lot more research in this area before any recommendations can be made regarding probiotics for ADHD. There are many strains of probiotics and we do not yet know which strains and in what amounts are the most helpful for ADHDers. Personally, I focus on eating plenty of fiber-rich foods (aka pre-biotics or what feeds the microbes in your gut) and fermented foods, such as yogurt or kimchi, to support my gut health.

The keto diet can also come with a number of adverse effects, including nutrient deficiencies, digestive issues, "keto flu" (headaches, brain fog, fatigue, irritability), kidney stones, fuzzy thinking and mood swings, and heart disease. This diet is contraindicated for folks with pancreatitis, liver failure, disorders of lipid metabolism, and those struggling with or who have a history of disordered eating or ED histories.

Due to the number of risks and there being no peer-reviewed research to support this diet for ADHD, I would not recommend trying it unless you are under the supervision of a dietitian or medical provider. I cannot stress enough that cutting out carbs is not a good idea if you have a history of disordered eating or binge eating. It will feed a binge/restrict cycle with carbs.

If you are thinking "But I eat too many carbs, feel addicted to them, etc.," stay tuned. We will talk more about how to approach your carb intake shortly.

Healthful Eating Patterns That Support ADHD Management

There are PLENTY of books that will tell you that if you eat a certain way, your ADHD will magically disappear. I completely understand wanting to find natural solutions to managing ADHD, but as we've seen, you cannot "cure" or "heal" ADHD with diet. *Period.* If you've tried any of the diets from the previous section and felt like a failure because your ADHD didn't go away, please know it was not your fault. Diet cannot change your genes or the structural differences seen in ADHD brains.

While no diet can "cause" or "cure" ADHD, how and what you eat can certainly impact the severity of your ADHD traits and your overall well-being. ADHDers tend to eat less healthful diets—meaning more added sugar, saturated fat, and sodium, typically from packaged foods, beverages, and eating at restaurants. These foods tend to be the focus of ADHDers's diets simply because they are easy sources of dopamine, they make it easier to avoid sensory sensitivities, and they provide quick energy for those who lack an appetite due to meds.

While there may not be a specific diet for ADHD, following a healthful eating pattern can help you feel better both mentally and physically. You may be familiar with MyPlate, which is a visual representation of the Dietary Guidelines for Americans. It recommends things like, "eat plenty of fruits and veggies, lean protein, limit added sugars, sodium, and saturated fats." You've probably heard messages like this more times than you can count, and your ADHD brain screams, "BORING!" because it's not novel or exciting advice. Fad diets are more exciting to us because they promise instant gratification or results or they (falsely) offer something "new" or "different." But often the reason you feel better on a new diet is because you are eating more fruits, vegetables, and lean proteins, and limiting added sugar, sodium, and saturated fat. The problem is that these fad diets are so

ADHD or Nutrient-Deficient?

If you correct nutrient deficiencies in your diet and you no longer experience ADHD traits, then the traits you were experiencing were a result of the nutrient deficiency and not ADHD. There are nutrient deficiencies that can mirror ADHD traits. For example, iron deficiency anemia can lead to fatigue, difficulty concentrating, and impaired cognitive function.

restrictive that they are not sustainable. If you can't eat that way for the rest of your life, the diet does not work for you. That's okay.

Two diets which may be helpful for ADHD are the Dietary Approaches to Stop Hypertension (DASH) and the Mediterranean diet. Both of these diets focus on generally healthful eating patterns, so let's chat about them and why they might be helpful for you.

Mediterranean Diet

Out of all of the "diets" that exist, the Mediterranean diet has been ranked the best overall diet by *U.S. News & World Report* for the past seven years. As a non-diet dietitian, I like this way of eating because there are no strict rules or complicated calculations required to determine what or how much to eat, nor are there any off-limits foods. Instead, it focuses on your overall eating patterns, which makes it a flexible and sustainable way of eating that aligns well with gentle nutrition. It highlights the importance of trying to eat more nutritious foods to support your ADHD brain.

Mediterranean diet principles include:

- Eating whole grains, fruits, vegetables, legumes, herbs, spices, nuts, and healthy fats daily
- Eating fish and seafood twice per week
- Consuming moderate portions of dairy, eggs, and poultry
- Limiting alcohol
- Regular social connection, like sharing meals, and movement

Children who follow this eating pattern tend to have the lowest risk of ADHD. This diet has also been shown to support cognitive improvements and mood disorders, particularly depression. This diet is higher in fiber and omega-3 fatty acids, which also benefit ADHD brains.

My only issue with this diet is that it is often presented as a whitewashed interpretation of the foods eaten in the Mediterranean region. Many other cultures eat fresh fruits and veggies, healthy fats, and fish. Just a reminder, you can still enjoy your cultural foods and eat healthfully.

DASH Diet—Dietary Approaches to Stop Hypertension

As the name implies, Dietary Approaches to Stop Hypertension (also called the DASH diet) is originally aimed at treating high blood pressure, but it is considered a healthy eating pattern for the general population as well. It focuses on eating the recommended amount of fiber and limiting sodium and added sugar intake. There's only one study on this diet, and it does show some positive results for those with ADHD.

Both this diet and the Mediterranean diet highlight how focusing on healthy dietary patterns will not only support ADHD but also support overall health. For this reason, it offers more helpful guidance than unsustainable elimination diets and supplements.

Bottom line? There's no denying that eating nutritious foods is important for our overall health and well-being and will help you feel better. But before we get into practical tools and strategies for gently incorporating more nutritious foods into your diet, let's talk about an important aspect of ADHD that often gets left out of the food conversation: sensory sensitivities.

Sensory Sensitivities are NOT Picky Eating

First off, let's drop the label "picky eater" for good. Everyone has food preferences or likes and dislikes with food. ADHDers can have stronger food preferences due to differences in sensory processing. This can lead to less variety in their diets. The label "picky eater" does more harm than good because it further stigmatizes food and eating habits, creates shame, and takes away from the complexity of eating challenges. We get enough of that in other areas of our lives! I'll be using terms such as selective eater and sensory sensitivities throughout this section to indicate that **your food preferences are valid.** I encourage you to do the same.

It's okay to have likes and dislikes with food. You do not need to eat every single food that exists or enjoy every way that a food is prepared. You don't have to eat certain foods just because everyone else tells you that you should or because they like them. Selective eaters often get told they "eat like a kid." If you like foods that society deems "kid" foods, that is okay.

It's important to accept and honor your own sensory preferences.

Common Sensory Sensitivities

There is a large variation in what foods ADHDers like and do not like. However, a few foods that are common sensory "icks" include eggs, yogurt, cottage cheese, chicken, fish, avocado, vegetables (especially mushy vegetables), and fruits. Unfortunately, many of these foods provide micronutrients that ADHDers need. Luckily, we can find these micronutrients in other foods.

Another problem for many ADHDers is that foods that give them an "ick" response can be consistently inconsistent. You might have a fried egg with breakfast every morning for three months, but suddenly one day you take a bite or look at it and your brain says "NOPE, can't eat that for a [insert unpredictable amount of time until you can eat it again]." This can be frustrating, but it's best to try and accept these ups and downs in the "ick" factor. When it happens, think about what type of nutrition this food provides and try exploring an alternative.

A big reason ADHDers—especially those with sensory sensitivities—tend to eat more processed foods is because they are consistent and predictable. When you open a package of food and take a bite, 99.9 percent of the time it will be what you expect it to be. This is not the case when it comes to eating whole foods, especially fruits and vegetables.

Hypo- vs. Hypersensitivities

If you have hyposensitivities to food, then you might seek out foods with lots of flavor, color, and more textures. If you have hypersensitivities to food, you might prefer blander, beige, and softer foods.

Fruits and Veggies

We all know that there are a lot of benefits to eating fruits and vegetables. Common nutrients in fruits and veggies include fiber, folate, vitamin C, vitamin K, iron, and potassium. Eating plenty of fruits and vegetables is linked to lowered blood pressure, reduced risk of heart disease and stroke, and more. Despite all the benefits of fruits and veggies, a 2019 study found that only 12.3 percent and 10.0 percent of adults surveyed met the recommended intakes for fruits and vegetables, respectively.

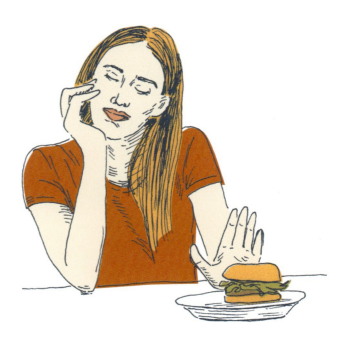

When It's More than "Picky Eating"

Avoidant Restrictive Food Intake Disorder, or ARFID, is a newer eating disorder that's "characterized as avoidance and aversion to food and eating," which leads to extreme selective eating. Unlike anorexia, ARFID is not rooted in a focus on body shape, size, or weight. It stems from a phobia or fear of food and/or fear of choking, vomiting, or getting sick from eating a food, increased sensitivity to sensory aspects of food, or a lack of interest in eating due to low appetite. ARFID is a serious eating disorder that can lead to malnutrition, significant weight loss, and inability to grow and maintain development in kids. ARFID, like all EDs, can really impact and interfere with your life because food is a big part of how we spend time with others.

It is estimated that up to 26 percent of people with ARFID also have ADHD. Most of the research around ARFID and treatment is focused on kids, but I suspect that as more adults get diagnosed with ADHD and autism, the rates for ARFID in adults will also increase.

Since this is a newer eating disorder, more research is needed to understand which treatments are most effective. Neurodiversity Affirming Model and Responsive Feeding Therapy are two treatment approaches often used. Both of these approaches are client centered and focus on accommodation and acceptance for feeding differences rather than trying to push someone with ARFID to meet "neurotypical" eating standards.

Like with all EDs, what recovery looks like is different for everyone, and it's vital to recovery for the goals created to be client centered. For a lot of ADHDers, recovery for ARFID may focus on restoring and maintaining your nutrition status versus aiming to eat a wide variety of foods.

One thing I find with veggies is that folks are afraid to make them taste good. Veggies do not need to be bland or boring for them to "count" as a vegetable. You can experiment with different herbs and spices, using different cooking methods like air frying, roasting, or grilling (these are all great if you like crispy or crunchy foods), using some fat in the cooking process, serving them with a dip, topping them with cheese, or drizzling them with honey. None of these things negate the nutrition that you get from these foods, and it means you'll get more of what you need.

If fruits are challenging for you, try squeeze pouches or frozen fruits. The texture and taste are more consistent and better in my opinion. Plus, you don't have to worry that they will go bad. I pour frozen blueberries in a bowl and eat them like fresh blueberries. I also like to do this with grapes, specifically cotton candy grapes, because it makes them like little popsicle bites.

Bottom line, it's worth experimenting to find at least a few fruits and veggies that you can at least tolerate. Learn what micronutrients they provide and look for other choices to add variety. Any way you can add them into your day is better than not having any.

Create a Safe Foods List

If you are a selective eater, it can be extremely helpful to create a list of your safe foods (and keep it visible). Include four main categories: anytime/preferred foods, sometimes/tolerable foods, going out foods, and foods you're curious about trying or have eaten in the past. You also may want a subcategory within each category to distinguish how long they take to make or how much executive function they use to make.

This is a flexible list, so if you find a new food you can add it or move foods around as needed.

It can be frustrating and challenging to navigate sensory sensitivities. Two mantras I find helpful are *fed is best* and *eating something is better than nothing*. These mantras may help you give yourself permission to eat something that may be less nutrient-dense to help you eat enough and regularly.

Gentle Nutrition in Your Daily Life

Now that we've debunked some myths about diets and ADHD and discussed some helpful strategies for dealing with sensory sensitivities, let's talk about applying gentle nutrition to your daily life.

In chapter 4, we discussed how the foundation of a healthy relationship with food is eating enough and eating regularly (about every three to four hours). Once you are able to do that *most of the time*, ditch restrictive dieting, and make peace with food, you can start to think about gentle nutrition. In Intuitive Eating this principle recommends making choices "that honor your health and taste buds while making you feel good." So gentle nutrition is all about combining pleasure, satisfaction, and health. Remember—your mental and emotional health are a part of your overall health.

I've said this several times but **fed is best.** I would much rather someone eat "too much" than not eat at all. If you struggle with meeting your energy needs, then the foods society labels "junk" may actually be necessary. This is why making peace with food is so important. You'll view all foods as morally and emotionally neutral. If your body is not getting enough energy, or calories, then you are more likely to experience low energy, fatigue, sleep disturbances, and feel moodier—all of which can impact your ADHD traits.

Restrictive diets usually remove pleasure and satisfaction from your eating, which can harm your mental and emotional health. You'll find you end up eating mostly nutritious foods because that's what makes you feel good. Again, this doesn't mean striving for perfection. It means making good enough choices based on your time, resources, cooking skills, and executive function.

Before we get into some specific principles and strategies, a quick disclaimer: the following section will include specific numbers, such as calories, grams of specific nutrients, etc. If you are currently struggling with or have a history of ED or disordered eating, you may want to skip this section for now.

Here are a few easy ways to start incorporating gentle nutrition into your daily life.

Focus on Addition, Not Subtraction

One good way to incorporate gentle nutrition into your life is to focus on addition, not subtraction. A popular mantra for this approach is **eat what you want and add what you need.** This can help not only limit feelings of deprivation, but it also encourages flexibility and balance in your eating pattern.

Adding more nutrient-dense foods to what you're eating can help you feel full for longer and promote a satisfying eating experience. Think about adding fiber from fruits and veggies, complex carbs, unsaturated fats, and lean protein to your meals. For example, try adding:

- Steamed broccoli (veg) and rotisserie chicken (protein) to mac and cheese
- Almond butter (fat), protein powder (protein), and blueberries (fruit) to oatmeal
- A side of carrots (veg) and ranch (fat) OR a salad (veg) with low-fat dressing as your side to pizza
- Chopped walnuts (fat) and sliced strawberries (fruit) to ice cream

Swap in More Nutrient-Dense Convenience Foods

Yes, some of these foods may be more expensive than the "original" version. The added cost or "ADHD tax" may feel worth it if you're thinking about your long-term health. Buy what you can afford and what works for your lifestyle. This is not necessarily about selecting a lower calorie option, but about selecting one that is going to provide you more bang for your buck in terms of the nutrients you get.

"Ultra-processed foods" get a bad rap because they tend to lack fiber and protein and they contain higher amounts of sodium, sugar, and saturated fats. If you have the budget to spend a little more to buy versions of foods you enjoy that are more nutrient-dense without sacrificing your enjoyment, this can be helpful. If something is your absolute favorite thing in the world and you don't really love the more nutrient-dense option that is okay.

Swaps my clients find helpful include:

- Protein or chickpea pasta for regular pasta
- Lower sugar probiotic soda or kombucha for soda
- Higher fiber, Higher protein bread for white bread
- Greek or Skyr for regular yogurt
- Protein chips or kale for potato chips
- Protein pancakes for regular pancakes
- Protein shake and cereal for milk and cereal
- Coffee with premade protein shake for coffee and creamer

How to Use a Food Label to Pick More Nutrient-Dense Options

Food labels can be a valuable tool if you are trying to decide between foods. The 5/20 Rule can help you with picking options that are more nutrient-dense. If the Daily Value (DV) percentage for a nutrient on the food label is 5 or less, then it is low in that nutrient. If the DV percentage is 20 or more, it is high in that nutrient. So you might look for something that is high in protein or fiber, but low in added sugars, sodium, or saturated fats.

Set Up Your Environment to Make It Easier to Make Healthful Choices

Our environment can influence our food choices. For ADHDers who struggle with traits like impulsivity or inattention, it's even more important to create an environment that helps you make healthful choices unconsciously. If you know you can be impulsive and are likely to grab something off the counter and eat without realizing it, you may want to keep hyperpalatable foods out of your immediate line of sight, like in your pantry. I am not saying hide them or ask someone to hide them because that won't work. But adding a barrier may help create enough space between your impulse and action to check in and ask yourself if that's what you truly want in that moment.

On the other hand, if you have more inattentive traits and forget to eat, then you would benefit from leaving some sort of nourishing food options out as a visual cue to eat. If your hunger is unpredictable or you are still learning those subtle cues, you might want to leave nuts, fruit squeeze pouches, protein powder or shakes, etc. in places where you spend a lot of time so food is accessible and you don't feel like you need to stop for fast food or candy at the gas station.

Don't Overcomplicate It

Before Intuitive Eating, my life revolved around micromanaging my food intake and movement. It prevented me from being present and enjoying life. Now, I don't live by "food rules." Instead I trust my body to tell me what, when, and how much to eat and have the tools to feed myself when my body is not being reliable.

It can be easy to overcomplicate nutrition because there's so much conflicting advice and nutrition is a complex science. But our bodies are really smart if we try to create space to listen to them.

It's okay if your plate looks like a "kid's plate" if it helps you get all the food groups. There's nothing wrong with simple meals. If your mom packed your lunch growing up, use that framework for simple lunches to bring to work. Check off a protein, a carb, a fat, a veggie, and a fruit. It's also okay if all of your meals don't contain every food group. Remember—*for the most part* you want to aim for all the food groups, but we aren't aiming for perfection. Sometimes you might not have a veggie on hand or you barely have an appetite so buttered noodles is the best you can do. That's okay.

Instead of getting caught up in the latest trend, get back to the basics of nutrition. Focus on:

- Eating enough
- Eating at regular intervals (every three to four hours)
- Developing other tools for regulation (both for stimulation and emotional regulation)

- Drinking mostly water
- Eating foods from all food groups (protein, carbs, fat, fruits, and veggies)
- Including foods you enjoy

You may notice that when you eat a more balanced diet, you may have more energy, a stabler mood, or better focus.

Limit Certain Foods If You Can

Saturated fat, sodium, and added sugar are three nutrients to consider limiting. Notice, I did not suggest "avoiding," "cutting out," or "eliminating" foods that contain these nutrients because, in reality, ADHDers are going to eat them. By "limiting," I mean aiming to follow the recommendations in the Dietary Guidelines for Americans (or your country's respective guidelines).

High intakes of saturated fat, sodium, and sugar are part of the standard American diet. You might notice eating them in excessive amounts doesn't make you feel good—physically or mentally. I fully embrace an all foods fit approach, but part of Gentle Nutrition is acknowledging that to some degree the foods we eat impact our health. When it comes to these three nutrients, all people—including ADHDers—could stand to be a little more mindful of their intake.

Swap Saturated Fat for Unsaturated Fats

Saturated fat is found mostly in animal-based fats with the exception of coconut oil and palm oil. It's considered an inflammatory fat. The recommendation for saturated fat is a maximum of 5 to 6 percent of total calories or about 12 grams saturated fat per day for a 2,000 calorie diet. Saturated fat is typically found in fattier cuts of meat, baked foods, fried foods, full-fat dairy, and butter. Try to swap saturated fats for unsaturated fats such as fatty fish, olive oil, avocados, nuts, and seeds. If you eat a lot of dairy, you may want to pick low-fat or fat-free versions.

Moderate Sodium Intake

Sodium or salt adds flavor and helps with the shelf-life of foods. Over 70 percent of the sodium in our diet comes from frozen foods, packaged foods, or food prepared outside your home. Consuming too much sodium can increase your risk for high blood pressure, heart disease, and stroke.

The average sodium intake in the United States is 3,500 milligrams per day. This is significantly higher than the American Heart Association's recommendation to consume less than 2,300 milligrams per day (1 teaspoon). When trying to reduce your sodium intake, look for packaged food options that are no sodium, low-sodium, reduced-sodium, or lightly salted. When cooking your own food, remember salt and pepper are not your only seasonings. Try seasoning your food with herbs and spices, like garlic, Italian seasoning, chili powder, or ginger instead.

Limit Added Sugars

Added sugar includes white sugar, honey, high-fructose corn syrup, agave, molasses, cane sugar, corn sweetener, raw sugar, fruit concentrates, and syrup. Sugar is added during the processing or preparation of foods to make it tastier. Sugar-sweetened beverages, candy, desserts, and sweet snacks are the biggest sources of added sugar. For example, one can of soda has 10 teaspoons or 39 grams of sugar!

Naturally occurring sugar found in milk, vegetables, or fruit are not the same thing. While all sugar gets broken down into glucose in the body, natural sugars also come with other nutrients like fiber, protein, and micronutrients. The fiber and protein help your body to more slowly absorb the sugar in these foods so your blood sugar will not respond with the same peak and crash that it gets from added sugar.

Food Labels and Sugar Content

Food packaging has very strict rules and requirements for how certain phrases are used. When it comes to sugar, there are several phrases and many of them can be confusing. Phrases like "reduced sugar," "lightly sweetened," "contains 30 percent less sugar" are unregulated terms that are often used to market something as "healthier," even if it isn't.

Here are some common terms and their definitions:

- Sugar-free: One serving contains less than 0.5 grams of sugar, both natural and added
- Reduced-sugar (less sugar, low in sugar, lower in sugar): Has at least 25 percent less sugar than the regular version of the product
- No sugar added (without added sugar or no sugar added): No sugar or ingredient containing sugar was added during processing or packaging.

The recommendation is to limit added sugar to less than 10 percent of your total calories. For a 2,000 calorie diet, this is about 12 tablespoons or 200 calories. For this reason, I view foods high in added sugar as play or fun foods instead of a primary source of energy or nutrition.

Non-nutritive sweeteners (NNS) or artificial sweeteners, like aspartame, saccharin, and sucralose, are alternatives to sugar that do not contain calories or sugar. These are considered "safe" if you stay below the acceptable daily intake (ADI). Sugar alcohols, like xylitol or erythritol, are another alternative. These provide less sweetness than NNS's and contribute to texture. They are often in a lot of diet foods such as protein shakes and bars as well as chewing gum. Novel sweeteners, like monk fruit and stevia, are "plant-derived natural sweeteners." They do not add significant calories, are less processed, and do not spike blood sugar like regular sugars. Some folks find these sweeteners are more similar in flavor to table sugar.

Focus on Building a Healthy Plate

Now that we've identified some nutrients that it can be helpful to limit, let's talk about what to include more of and how to create a nourishing plate. In this section, we'll review some nutrition basics and why they are important for ADHD brains.

As mentioned earlier, MyPlate is a visual representation of the Dietary Guidelines for Americans. These guidelines are created based on current peer-reviewed science to "promote health, reduce risk of chronic disease, and meet nutrients needs" and updated every five years. **It's estimated that only 10 percent of adults in the United States meet these guidelines.**

The emphasis of MyPlate is to pick nutrient-dense foods from each of the following categories: vegetables, fruits, grains, dairy, protein foods, and oil. A healthful eating pattern includes foods from all of these groups. This means including all macronutrients—carbohydrates, fat, and protein—in your eating pattern, each of which serves different functions in our bodies (more on this in the next section). I recommend aiming for all three macronutrients at meals and at least two of the three for snacks.

When building a meal, MyPlate recommends that:

- ½ your plate = fruits and/or veggies
- ¼ your plate = varied protein sources
- ¼ your plate = grains with at least half being whole grains
- Include low-fat dairy or fortified soy alternatives for calcium and vitamin D
- Limit added sugars, saturated fat, sodium, and alcohol intake

Where IE may differ from MyPlate is including the satisfaction factor in our eating experiences. For me, the satisfaction factor can be a few things: what gets me excited about the meal, a flavor, a texture, an aroma, or creating an enjoyable eating environment. It can be anything from adding Everything Bagel Seasoning to my avocado toast, focusing on the crispy texture and taste of roasted garlic potatoes, or enjoying my lunch on the balcony with my dogs. I try to include these things in my eating experience as often as possible. If I cannot for whatever reason, I aim for fed is best with as many of these things as I can manage at the time.

If you're overwhelmed at the idea of getting your plate to look like this, I totally get it! You can focus on small changes and work your way up. I don't expect you to do this overnight so be patient and curious so you can figure out what works for you. In the next chapter, we will discuss strategies to ease overwhelm around cooking so it's easier to make a plate like this.

Now that we've covered some basic ways of incorporating gentle nutrition into your daily life, let's take a deeper dive into some specific aspects of nutrition for ADHD.

Understanding Macronutrients

When my clients are ready to start learning about gentle nutrition, we start by focusing on two nutrients: protein and fiber. This can be a great strategy if MyPlate feels too overwhelming or confusing for you at the beginning. But before you can start adding more protein and fiber into your diet, you need to understand what they are and what they do in your body. So let's talk more about macronutrients—carbohydrates, protein, and fat.

Carbs

Carbs are probably the most demonized macronutrient, despite it being our body's preferred and primary source of energy. Your body breaks down carbs into glucose (sugar). You can think of glucose as the gas that makes your engine, or metabolism, function. Your stomach, intestine, liver, kidneys, gallbladder, and muscles are all involved in regulating your blood sugar or glucose levels. Your brain, red blood cells, and nerve cells primarily rely on glucose to function properly.

While protein always gets pushed as the most important macronutrient for ADHD brains, it's important to realize that glucose is the primary energy source for your brain. It is so important that if your glucose levels fall below ~40mg/dL, it can cause permanent brain damage and even death. During fasting, starvation, or doing a diet low in carbs, your body will breakdown fat into ketone bodies to supply your brain with energy. It's a backup system that our bodies developed to protect us during periods of starvation but is not intended to be a long-term source of fuel for our bodies.

When you consume more carbs than your cells need, your body stores glucose in your muscle so it can use it during periods of fasting and high-intensity exercise. Can you eat too many carbs? Of course you can. Eating too much of anything will probably not make you feel great. Many people fear carbs because they think simply eating any carbs will lead to weight gain. But this is not true. Eating more energy than your body burns, regardless of if its form, will lead to weight gain. But eating a banana, having a sandwich with whole-grain bread, or enjoying pasta doesn't automatically turn into body fat.

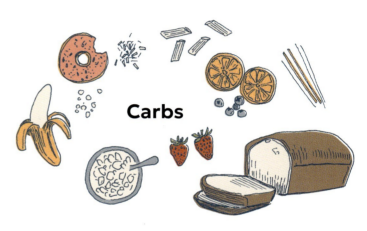

You do not need to fear carbs. Some carbs may be more nutrient-dense than others, but they can all fit into a healthful eating pattern, including foods like cookies or ice cream. So let's talk about the different types of carbs.

Simple vs. Complex Carbs

Instead of "good" and "bad" carbs, think of them as complex and simple carbs. When someone says something is a "good" carb, they are referring to carbs that contain fiber such as fruits, brown rice, beans, corn, peas, potatoes, oatmeal, quinoa, high-fiber cereals, and breads. Complex carbs take longer to digest, so they lead to a more gradual increase in blood sugar and provide more stable energy. "Bad" carbs are often simple carbs that are high in sugar and lack fiber, like fruit juice, white bread, white rice, pasta, candy, chips, etc. Think of simple carbs as quick energy. They can spike your blood sugar higher and faster. BUT you can pair them with a fat and/or protein to help slow that down.

MyPlate recommends aiming for about half of your carbs to be complex carbs. This is because they contain more fiber and micronutrients. So, if you feel like you are addicted to carbs or out of control around carbs, reflect on what kinds of carbs you are eating. Are you eating mostly simple carbs? If you said yes, try focusing on ways you can swap them for more fiber-rich carb sources and take note of how you feel. When my clients focus on ADDING enough complex carbs to meet the recommendation for fiber, they find they don't crave sugar as much. This is likely because their body is getting the energy it needs from complex carbs. If you are someone who is constantly trying to restrict carbs only to find yourself binge eating them, you can also try focusing on eating enough complex carbs. This means including them at your meals and snacks.

Simple carbs without fiber or micronutrients can still fit into a healthful eating pattern. Remember **all foods can fit.** When your blood sugar is low, simple carbs are actually the better choice because they are more easily digested so you can get quick energy. This is why it's important to have flexibility and be able to adapt to what your body needs in that moment.

Simple carbs are also fun foods that may be more nourishing to our souls by providing comfort or the chance to connect with others, like grabbing a coffee and a pastry with a friend. Sometimes you might be in a situation where simple carbs are your only accessible source of

dopamine—and that's okay too. Just consider pairing them with a fat or protein if you want to feel full for longer.

Fiber

Fiber is one of the two nutrients I encourage my clients to focus on getting enough of. Unless you have Crohn's and benefit from a low-fiber diet, fiber is your friend. Eating enough fiber is important for regular bowel movements (unless you have conditions like Crohn's disease) and blood sugar regulation, helps feed the microbes in your gut to support your gut health, lowers cholesterol, reduces your risk of colorectal cancer, and more.

There are two types of fiber: insoluble fiber and soluble fiber. Insoluble fiber helps move material through your GI tract and provides bulk for your stool. Soluble fiber creates more of a gel. Eating a variety of plant foods can help you get both types of fiber.

If you don't eat a lot of fiber in your current diet, then it is recommended to gradually increase your fiber intake to avoid gas, bloating, and cramping.

Fiber Recommendations Include:

- Women ages 19-50: 25g/day
- Women ages 51+: 21g/day
- Men ages 19-50: 38g/day
- Men ages 51+: 30g/day

High-Fiber Foods Include:

- Ground flaxseed
- Chia seeds
- Berries: Raspberries, blueberries, blackberries, strawberries
- Apples
- Avocado
- Artichokes
- Brussels sprouts
- Sweet potato and potatoes
- Oatmeal
- Lentils
- Quinoa
- Beans: black, pinto, lima, white, navy, kidney
- Chickpeas
- Low-carb wraps
- Barley
- High-fiber bread
- Lentil or chickpea pasta

Protein

Many ADHDers don't get enough protein. This is due to our preference for carbs, as they are more accessible, affordable, provide a quick source of dopamine, and are common safe foods if you have sensory sensitivities. Plus, carbs are delicious.

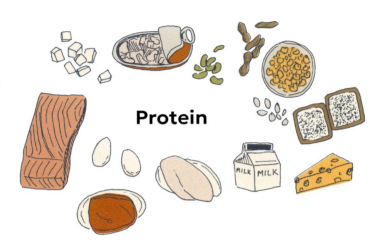

Protein

But protein is important for ADHDers. It functions as the building blocks for many things in our bodies. Protein does not get stored in the body to the same degree as fat and carbs. This is one reason it is important to regularly consume protein throughout your day. Another reason is that protein helps stimulate the production of leptin, which is a hormone that helps signal fullness in your stomach.

Protein is made of amino acids, which are the building blocks for neurotransmitters, like dopamine. In theory, eating more protein will help increase the production of neurotransmitters like dopamine. However, to date there not any studies that specifically focus on high vs. low protein diets for ADHD. Even so, both my clients and myself have found that increasing protein intake can be helpful.

Protein needs depend on age, activity levels, and other factors (like if you are breastfeeding). For most folks, the recommendation for protein is 0.8 grams to 1.2 grams of protein per kilogram of body weight. If you are not eating enough protein, aim for the minimum of 0.8 grams per kilogram of body weight to start. Generally, this means:

- Aim for 20 grams of protein at meals
- Aim 10 to 15 grams of protein at snacks

For most people, these amounts will help you achieve a high-protein diet. Examples of foods with at least 20 grams protein include an average sized chicken breast, single-serve Greek yogurt, single-serve low-fat cottage cheese, protein shake, lean beef patty, chicken sausage, tofu, lentils, or a can of tuna.

Fat

Fat is the most energy-dense macronutrient at 9 calories per gram, so our bodies need the least amount of it. It takes the longest to digest out of the three macronutrients, which means it plays a big role in helping you feel full and satisfied. It also enhances the flavor and texture of food.

Fat plays an important role in our nervous system, and in producing and regulating hormones, like estrogen. It is required for absorbing fat-soluble vitamins (vitamins A, D, E, K) and helps improve the asorption of phytochemicals, which are health-promoting chemicals found in fruits and vegetables. Even body fat has the function of providing insulation and protection for your organs.

There are two main types of fat: saturated fats and unsaturated fats. A third type of fat, trans fat, has been eliminated from the US food supply. Although, I don't like using "healthy" vs. "unhealthy" labels to describe food, I am going to in reference to fat because that is the common language used. There are healthy fats and unhealthy fats. Let's take a look at both.

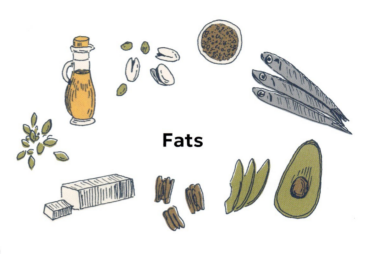

Fats

- Beef
- Pork
- Coconut
- Palm and palm kernel oil
- Ice cream
- Cream
- Baked and fried foods

Saturated Fats

Saturated fats are often referred to as "unhealthy fats." Saturated fats tend to come from animal products, like fatty cuts of meat and butter, with the exception of coconut oil, palm oil, and palm kernel oil. Saturated fats can increase your LDL (bad) cholesterol, which can form plaque in your arteries and increase your risk for heart disease and stroke. Aim to swap saturated fats for unsaturated fats, especially polyunsaturated fats, as much as possible.

Saturated fats are often solid at room temperature. Common sources include:

- Butter
- Frozen meals
- Pizza
- Full-fat dairy including cheese
- Skin on chicken or turkey

Unsaturated Fats

Unsaturated fats are often referred to as "healthy" fats because higher intakes are associated with improved blood cholesterol, decreased inflammation, stabilized heart rhythms and other benefits. These fats are mostly found in plants, like vegetable oils, nuts, and seeds, as well as fish. They are liquid at room temperature. Most people do not consume enough of these fats, so it can be helpful to try to swap saturated fats for unsaturated fats as much as possible. There are two forms of this fat: monounsaturated and polyunsaturated fats (PUFAs). Note that PUFAs contain both Omega 3s and Omega 6s, which are essential fatty acids that we must get through food because our bodies cannot make them.

Type of Unsaturated Fats	What They Do	Sources
Monounsaturated Fats	Play a role in developing and maintaining your cells	Nuts such as cashews, almonds, peanuts, pecans, seeds like sunflower and pumpkin seeds, avocado, canola oil, olive oil, safflower oil, sunflower oil, peanut oil, sesame oil
Polyunsaturated Fats (PUFAs)	Contains omega-3 and omega-6 fatty acids, which are important for brain health and cell growth	Walnuts, flaxseed or flaxseed oil, chia seeds, corn oil, soybean oil, safflower oil, and fish such as salmon, tuna, mackerel, trout, or herring

Eating Enough—Calories That Is

All three macronutrients provide energy or calories. When I say it's important to eat "enough," that means eating enough calories or energy. So, how much is enough?

The amount of energy or calories your body needs will depend on your age, gender, and activity level. If you've dieted, the number of calories you think you need may be extremely skewed because most diets do not provide adequate calories for an adult. (Consuming fewer calories also makes it really hard to meet your micronutrient needs.) For example, most calorie counting apps will set the calorie needs to lose weight for a woman at 1,200 calories, which is the minimum amount of calories recommended for kids ages 5 to 8.

Estimated Energy Needs for Adults

Gender and Age	Calorie Needs
Females ages 19-30	1,800-2,400 calories per day
Females ages 31+	1,600-2,200 calories per day
Males ages 19-30	2,400-3,000 calories per day
Males ages 31-59	2,200-3,000 calories per day
Males ages 60+	2,200-2,600 calories per day

For trans and non-binary folks, it's recommended to follow the recommendation of your biological sex assigned at birth.

For pregnant and lactating folks, energy needs will be higher.

If you are unsure about how much food you should be eating, please consult with a dietitian to ask the calorie range to aim for to maintain weight.

Hopefully, this section has helped you better understand the three macronutrients and how to incorporate them into your diet. For the final section in this chapter, I'm going to provide my thoughts on a topic you've probably heard a lot of buzz about in the ADHD world: supplements.

Supplements for ADHD

Most people assume because I am a dietitian who works with ADHDers, that I recommend taking a bunch of supplements for ADHD. I think supplements are great to correct nutrient deficiencies and fill in nutritional gaps. But taking supplements is not the same as getting these nutrients from food and nowhere near as effective as stimulant medications when it comes to ADHD management. **You cannot supplement your way out of a poor diet.**

Many supplements are marketed for ADHD. Most have not been well studied, if studied at all. In this section we will review some common supplements recommended for ADHD, the research behind them, and ways to incorporate foods rich in these micronutrients as an alternative.

Pros and Cons of Supplements

There are over 100,000 dietary supplements available to consumers. The only time I recommend supplements for my clients is when they are not getting enough of an essential nutrient or there is strong peer-reviewed research to support using them for a specific condition. As stated earlier in this chapter, there is not enough research to support using micronutrients or probiotics in the management of ADHD. So I take a food first approach and try to find ways to make it easier to get in more whole foods.

That being said, some benefits to taking supplements include:

- Bridging nutritional gaps
- Correcting specific nutrient deficiencies
- Convenience
- Enhanced sports performance
- May help with disease prevention

Supplements are often viewed as safer because they are more "natural" than medication. But supplements still come with risks. Supplements are not regulated, so manufacturers can make false claims to profit off of your health fears and insecurities. When it comes to ADHD, this includes many supplements that are unnecessary and haven't been studied.

Some of the cons of supplements include:

- Lack of regulation
- Unwanted side effects: Liver damage, increased risk of bleeding, and nervous system damage
- Negative interactions with medications and other supplements
- Risk for toxicity and overdosing
- Quality concerns: May contain impurities, contaminants, and labels may be inaccurate
- Can be expensive

Always talk to your doctor before starting a supplement, especially if you take medications. Supplements can interact with each other and other medications you take, which can be dangerous.

Multivitamins
Multivitamins are not recommended to manage ADHD, but you may want to consider taking one if you don't eat a lot of fruits and veggies, your diet lacks variety, or you struggle with eating enough.

Commonly Recommended Supplements for ADHD and What the Research Says

St. John's Wort

St. John's Wort is an herb that may increase the availability of neurotransmitters like dopamine, similar to some antidepressants. It has a lot of *significant interactions* with other supplements and medications and has been shown to be no more effective than a placebo for ADHD.

L-tyrosine

Found in protein sources, L-tyrosine is an amino acid that is the precursor for dopamine, which ADHDers crave, epinephrine, and norepinephrine. Studies have shown it has benefits for neurological conditions such as Parkinson's disease, but there are zero studies on it for ADHDers at the time of this writing.

Since you can find L-tyrosine in protein-rich foods, this is a better way to go. The money you would spend on a supplement every month could be put towards buying higher quality proteins such as grass-fed beef or wild-caught fish.

Nootropics

Nootropics are compounds or supplements that enhance cognitive performance. These include stimulant drugs as well as supplements. The most effective nootropics are stimulant drugs, like Adderall and Ritalin, as well as nonstimulant drugs like Modafinil. These outperform all the other types of nootropics when it comes to executive function. Additionally, these drugs have extensive research to support their safety and efficacy and are highly regulated.

Nootropic supplements are a very different story. These can be a single-ingredient supplement or a "stack," which is a blend of micronutrients, botanicals, and other nutrients that have been studied for ADHD or cognitive performance. These supplements carry the risk for potential interactions with medications because they contain many different ingredients, and they can contain ingredients not listed on the label.

Companies that sell these nootropic "stacks" are excellent at marketing, use fear of pharmaceuticals, and perpetuate harmful stereotypes around stimulants (like equating them to hard drugs), so be cautious. They will cite research looking at a single-ingredient nootropic as evidence for their supplement. But there is no guarantee that when combined with other ingredients, that nootropic will have the same effect, which is why we have clinical trials. None of the supplemental nootropics have well-designed clinical trials with large sample sizes so there is not nearly as much evidence to support their long-term safety and efficacy.

Magnesium

Research shows ADHDers are more likely to have lower magnesium levels in their blood. Magnesium is a mineral that comes in many forms and each has a different purpose. L-threonate is the form of magnesium that is being studied for ADHD, with promising results, though we don't have enough research yet to establish a therapeutic dose for ADHD.

It is possible to take too much magnesium in supplement form, but this isn't the case with magnesium from food sources, so I recommend getting it that way. Nuts and seeds are the richest sources of magnesium, but dark leafy greens, legumes, and whole grains are also great sources.

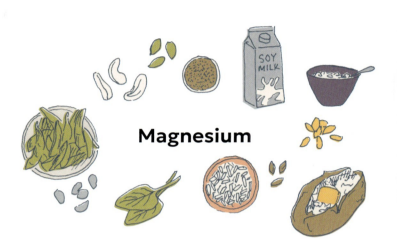

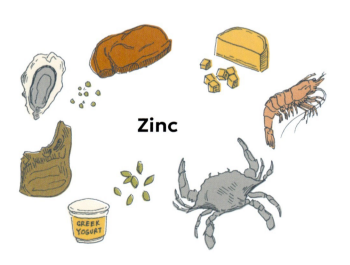

Zinc

Zinc is another mineral that ADHDers may have lower levels of and has been studied as a supplement to manage ADHD. A systematic review and dose-response meta-analysis rated the certainty of evidence for zinc supplementation as moderate to very low for all outcomes.

Zinc deficiency can cause loss of appetite and interfere with taste and smell. So if you don't eat a lot of zinc-rich foods and have a lot of sensory sensitivities, it might be worth trying to eat more. Oysters are the best source. You can also get it from beef, pork, and poultry. You can also find zinc in beans, nuts, and whole grains, but our bodies absorb less of the mineral from these plant sources.

Iron

Lower concentrations of iron in the brain may be linked to ADHD. Iron is frequently studied with zinc and may be helpful for a subset of youths with ADHD. Iron comes in two forms: heme iron and non-heme iron. Heme iron is found in animal sources and non-heme iron is found in plant sources. Humans are not great at absorbing non-heme iron so it is recommended to pair non-heme iron sources with vitamin C-rich foods listed in the following section to increase the absorption.

Lean meats and seafood are the best sources of heme iron. You can also find it in beans, dark leafy greens, and fortified grains.

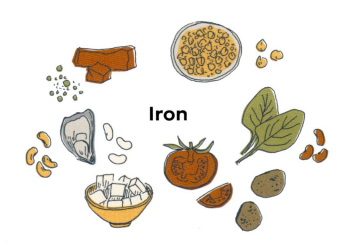

Iron

Vitamin C

Vitamin C appears to be involved in dopamine production, but we do not fully understand its role yet. High doses of vitamin C (>1,000mg) can interact with amphetamine-based ADHD meds, so if you are taking a high dose (for example, from an immune supplement like Emergen-C), you need to wait to take it an hour before or after taking your ADHD meds so that your body can absorb all of your medication.

The best source of vitamin C is fruits and vegetables. Some vitamin C can be lost via cooking and prolonged storage. Luckily, steaming and microwaving can reduce some of the losses and many fruits and veggies rich in vitamin C can be eaten raw.

B Vitamins

There are eight different B vitamins. Researchers have identified several B vitamins that ADHDers have lower levels of compared to individuals without ADHD. These include riboflavin (B2), vitamin B6, folate (B9), and vitamin B12.

B vitamins are involved in regulating energy and producing neurotransmitters. Riboflavin (B2) helps with the growth, development, and function of cells as well as converting food into energy. Riboflavin can be found in eggs, organ meats, lean meats, milk, mushrooms, quinoa, and bagels.

Vitamin B6 is involved in forming dopamine. The richest sources are fish, beef liver, potatoes, chickpeas, and non-citrus fruits. B6 is also found in a wide variety of foods such as dark leafy greens, fruits, fruit juices, nuts, beans, peas, seafood, eggs, dairy, meat, poultry, and fortified grains.

Folate (B9) is needed to synthesize DNA and neurotransmitters. Folate is found in beef liver, spinach, black-eyed peas, fortified breakfast

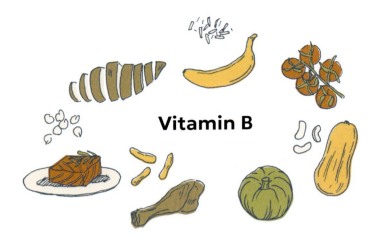

Vitamin B

cereals, rice, asparagus, Brussels sprouts, enriched pasta, romaine lettuce, avocado, and spinach.

Vitamin B12 is important for the health of your red blood cells and nerve cells, and plays a role in DNA synthesis. You can find vitamin B12 in beef liver, clams without shells, oysters, nutritional yeast, salmon, tuna, beef, 2% milk, yogurt, and fortified breakfast cereals.

Fish Oil

Fish oil is an excellent source of omega-3 fatty acids. Omega-3 fatty acids from foods can support brain health, but it is unclear whether the supplemental form boosts brain health and optimizes cognitive function. This is probably the most widely researched and recommended supplement for ADHD, though the findings show marginal to nonexistent efficacy in helping with ADHD symptoms.

If you do want to try it, look for a fish oil supplement that has 1.5 to 2 times more EPA than DHA and that is third-party tested.

Remember, Gentle Nutrition is about getting the pendulum to stop swinging between the extremes of undereating or being overly restrictive and overeating, bingeing, or eating

whatever you want, regardless of how it makes you feel.

Focus on eating enough, eating regularly, and making peace with food before you try to incorporate Gentle Nutrition. Your ADHD brain might want to overhaul your diet and change everything all at once, but that rarely leads to sustainable behavior change. Remember to be kind and patient with yourself on your journey, and that progress wins over perfection.

Now that we've talked about the importance of getting the right nutrients to support your ADHD brain, let's talk about HOW you can do that in a way that works for you. That means it's finally time to get cooking!

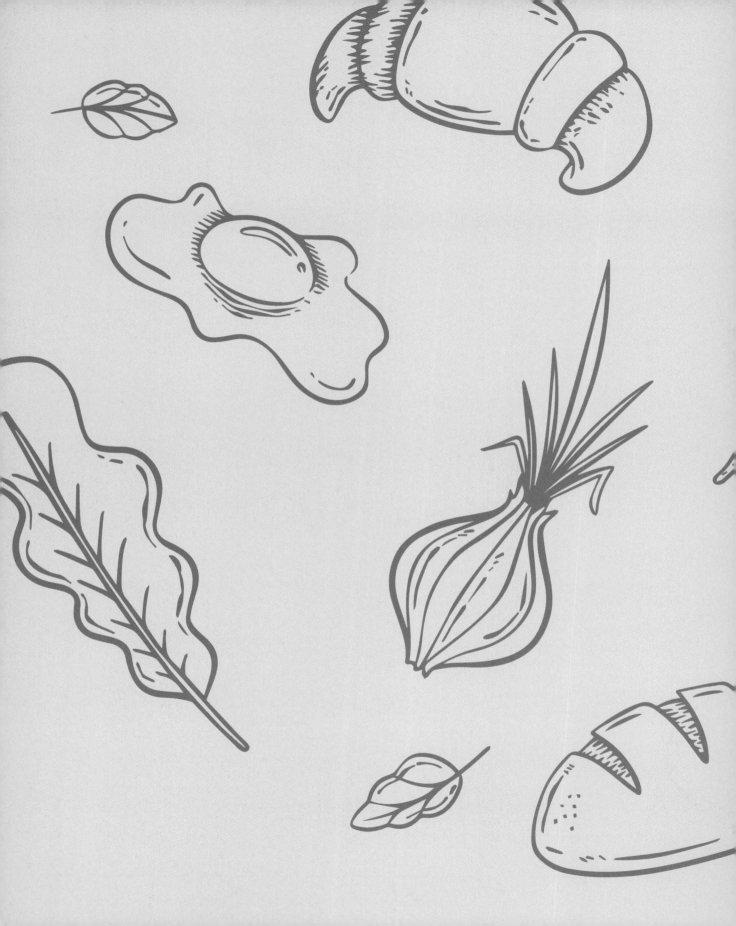

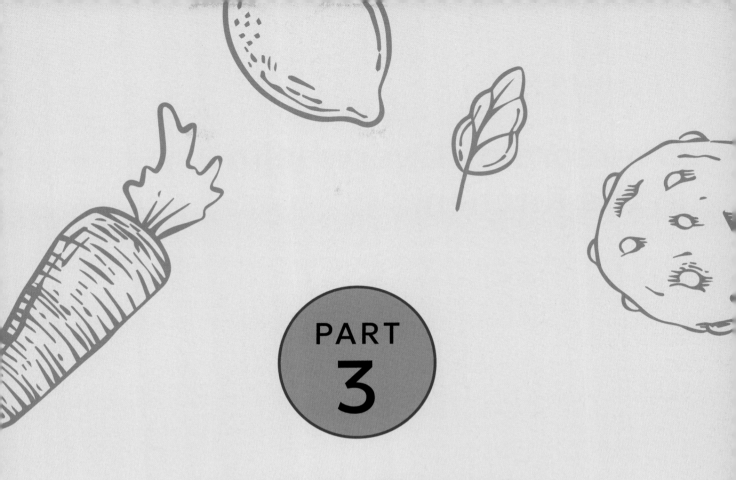

PART
3

Let's Get Cooking!

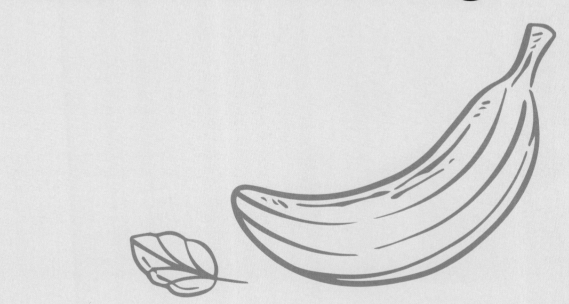

CHAPTER 8

Overcoming Overwhelm in the Kitchen

When you have ADHD, every step of cooking can feel HUGE. Deciding what to eat, getting all the ingredients, prepping and cooking, and then dealing with the cleanup; all of these steps might feel so overwhelming that you avoid the executive task of cooking until you're super hungry. At that point, you might say "screw it" and spend way too much on takeout again or opt for a bag of potato chips instead of eating the meal you planned.

One of the most common statements I hear from ADHDers is "I know what I 'should' be eating, but I can't figure out how to do it." I hear from so many ADHDers who want to cook more, eat more fruits and veggies, spend less money on fast food or takeout, but figuring out how to do that consistently is too overwhelming. Fortunately, there are many tools and strategies you can use to make feeding yourself a little easier. The goal of this chapter is to help you identify areas of overwhelm and/or barriers to cooking and explore strategies that work with

your ADHD brain to reduce those barriers, so you can cook more and maybe even find joy in the process. To do this, we're going to break down "making a meal" into each of its individual steps and discuss strategies for each of them. The steps are:

- Meal Planning
- Grocery Shopping
- Kitchen Organization
- Food Prep
- Cooking
- Cleanup

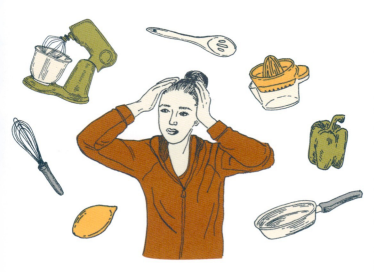

One of the big things to remember is that **there is no one "right" way to do any of these steps.** (Except for certain cooking methods and rules, like cooking meat, poultry, and fish to certain temperatures to prevent foodborne illnesses.) I want you to let go of the idea that you "should" do these steps a certain way or that you "should" do every single step in this process. It's okay if all of these steps feel HUGE and overwhelming. You wouldn't be reading this book if you found them easy. Get curious and figure out what works best for you and your brain.

Ready to get cooking? We'll start with meal planning.

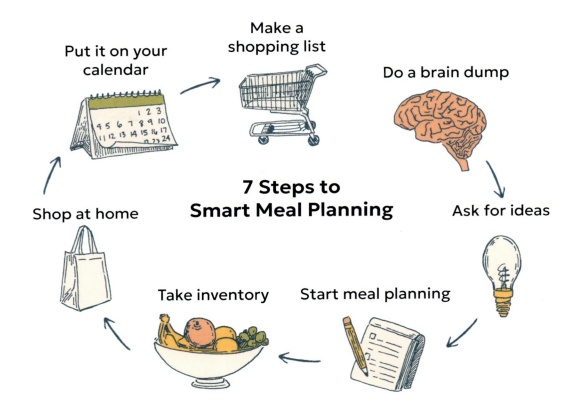

7 Steps to Smart Meal Planning

Put it on your calendar → Make a shopping list → Do a brain dump → Ask for ideas → Start meal planning → Take inventory → Shop at home

Meal Planning

It's easier to initiate the task of preparing food if you have an idea ahead of time about what you might make or what options you have on hand. That means meal planning. I wish I could say there is one method for meal planning that works for all ADHDers, but we all have different lifestyles, cooking skills, food access, etc., so that's unrealistic. You will likely need to use different meal planning strategies throughout your life, depending on your schedule or the season of life you're in. You might have to have a strategy for low executive function weeks and another for high executive function weeks. Not every strategy in this section will be needed or will work for you.

Meal planning typically involves deciding what you are going to eat for a certain period of time. I like to think of meal planning as a flexible framework for making grocery shopping and cooking easier. It is helpful to do some sort of planning before you shop so you have an idea of what to get and what you will likely make that week.

Common meal planning challenges for ADHDers include:

- Remembering to do it
- Setting aside enough time to sit and plan
- Not sure how to get started
- Feeling overwhelmed
- Your preferences might change so it's hard to plan
- You plan but struggle with executing what you planned
- You don't have the energy to make what you planned

In this section we're going to discuss strategies to help you overcome these challenges: how to decide what to eat in the moment, barriers to meal planning, strategies for meal planning, meal and snack formulas, and tools for meal planning.

Before we get started, though, here are some questions I want you to consider:

- Do you have a current strategy for meal planning? If so, what is it? What parts of this strategy work for you and what parts don't work?
- Do you make any meals at home? Which meals? How often?
- How many meals can you realistically prepare or cook per week right now?
- What is the maximum amount of time you want to spend cooking?
- Are there days of the week you know you will not have the energy or time to prepare meals?

- What is your typical eating pattern like? Do you typically eat out on the weekends?
- Would meal planning be approachable if you only planned for the workweek (Monday through Friday) and left the weekends open?
- Are you doing all of the cooking or do you share this responsibility with a partner, roommate, etc.?
- What is your goal with meal planning?

To make the most out of the next sections, I'd encourage you to set a timer for 20 minutes and answer the questions above. Answering these questions is kind of like surveying land before you build on it. It will be a lot easier to try implementing new strategies and tools if you have an idea of where you're starting from.

The Basics: How Do I Make a Meal Plan?

Now that you've spent some time thinking about how meal planning fits into your life, let's start with the basics of how to make one. It's often hard for ADHDers to plan out what they're going to eat because their preferences can be unpredictable. Our need for novelty and impulsivity, and perception of time as "now" versus "not now" can make figuring out what you're going to eat in the future tough.

But that does not mean that you can't make a meal plan. It just means a rigid meal planning style doesn't work for you. Rigid meal planning involves picking your meals and assigning when you will eat them. If that doesn't work for you, trying to force it will likely cause guilt, add unnecessary friction, and make cooking harder.

Instead, consider adding flexibility to your meal planning. Flexible meal planning removes the self-imposed rule of assigning a day to eat each meal. Instead, you select the meals you want to make for the week, but don't assign the days you'll eat them. This leaves room for spontaneity and your changing preferences. It also meshes well with Intuitive Eating.

Meal Planning, Step 1: Establish When You will Meal Plan

If you are going to make a meal plan, you need to have time set aside to do it. At a bare minimum, establish a day for meal planning (note: meal planning is different than meal prepping, where you make a bunch of food in advance, a strategy which doesn't work for a lot of ADHDers). Consider getting more specific by picking a time of the day like Saturday mornings or choosing a specific time by which it has to be done (i.e., noon on Saturday). This can give you some flexibility, but there is a deadline. Also remember, there might be weeks when you don't get to meal planning that day and that is okay.

If you have unpredictable preferences, you might benefit from planning and shopping for a few days at a time (more on this in the next step). This would mean meal planning and grocery shopping more than once a week.

Meal Planning, Step 2: Determine How Many Meals and Snacks You Need to Plan and Work Backward

Start with how many meals and snacks you will eat across your given time and then work backwards to fill them in. A typical eating pattern is three meals and two snacks per day. That means for a whole week of eating, you would need to plan out 21 meals and 14 snacks. Does that feel like a lot of planning?

If so, would meal planning be approachable if you only planned for the work week (Monday through Friday) and left the weekends open (so you're planning 15 meals and 10 snacks)? Some things to keep in mind when you're thinking about this: how many meals can you realistically cook? How many days can you eat leftovers? How many meals do you plan to eat out or get delivery/takeout? Do you pack your lunch? Are there any meals or snacks you eat on repeat or automate?

Meal Planning, Step 3: Evaluate Meals and Snacks Based on Nutrition and Satisfaction Needs and Tweak Accordingly

When you plan a meal, there are five components you want to aim to include: protein, carbohydrates, fat, fruits/veggies, and the satisfaction factor.

In the chapter on Gentle Nutrition, I discussed in-depth why these components are important. *For the most part*, you want to include all five components to have a satisfying and satiating meal. It's okay if 100 percent of your meals don't look like this, but it's worth reviewing your meal plan and tweaking your meals to get a few more of these components in where you can.

Here are a few meals that follow this formula:

- **Breakfast:** 2 fried eggs + 2 slices high-fiber bread + avocado + berries + everything bagel seasoning
- **Lunch:** deli turkey + bread + cheese (sandwich), apple, dark chocolate square
- **Dinner:** tofu + rice + sesame oil + frozen stir-fry veggie mix + soy sauce + sriracha

Snacks can be a great tool to incorporate more fruits and vegetables into your diet. For filling snacks, ideally you want to try to include two of your three macronutrients: Carb + fat OR Carb + Protein OR Protein + Fat.

I highly recommend low-effort snacks and grab and go snacks. Snacks don't need to be complicated. It is important to have snacks that are accessible so you can honor your hunger and save spoons for other tasks including cooking. The less time you spend making a snack the more time you have to enjoy that snack.

Snack examples:

- Snack packs with nuts, cheese, and dried fruit
- Tuna pouch + high-fiber crackers
- Apple + peanut butter or sunflower butter (nut-free)
- Dry roasted edamame + sunflower seeds
- Greek or coconut-based yogurt + blueberries
- Ready to drink protein shake
- Fruit squeeze pouch + high-fiber granola bar
- Cottage cheese + pineapple
- Potato chips + jerky

Meal Planning: Real-Life Example

Here is a summary of my meal planning process for you to use as an example. I typically eat some version of eggs, toast with a spread (avocado, cottage cheese, almond butter with jam) and fruit or some version of oatmeal if I need a quick breakfast (that takes care of 7 meals). I don't plan for Saturdays or Sundays because I usually eat out, order takeout, eat leftovers, or get motivated to cook something (4 meals and 4 snacks). So, I only have to plan 10 meals and 10 snacks.

Some of my typical snacks are carrots and a dip, apple, cheese, granola bar, cottage cheese, nuts and Greek yogurt with berries. These are safe foods in the sense that I know I can eat them on my meds, they meet my sensory preferences, they are all grab and go, and I can mix and match them based on what sounds good. So there is some flexibility.

I have learned I can actively cook at least three dinners each week. So I use a meal kit that comes with three meals and two servings for each so that covers six meals. Now, all that is left is four meals. It usually breaks down to two lunches and two dinners. These four meals are either a smoothie, frozen meal, veggie wrap with chips, salad kit with frozen grilled chicken and a carb that sounds good, or soup and salad with bread. So, when I go to the store, I only have to shop for cooking basics (cooking spray, minced garlic), snacks, breakfast food items, fruits, a frozen meal or two, and vegetables. Remember that what you eat is going to be unique to you and your needs.

Meal	Mon	Tues	Wed	Thurs	Fri	Sat	Sun
Meal #1	Avocado toast, egg, fruit	Cottage cheese toast, egg, fruit	Cottage cheese toast, egg, fruit	Oatmeal with berries and peanut butter	Cottage cheese toast, egg, fruit	Avocado toast, egg, fruit	Avocado toast, egg, fruit
Meal #2	Chicken salad wrap, sliced peppers, chips	Leftover tofu stir-fry	Leftover sheet pan meal	Leftover shrimp tostadas	Smoothie	X	X
Meal #3	Tofu stir-fry	Chicken sausage, sweet potato, and veggie sheet pan meal	Shrimp tostadas	Frozen meal	Tomato soup, side salad, and whole wheat bread	X	X

Snack	Mon	Tues	Wed	Thurs	Fri	Sat	Sun
Snack #1	Apple and cheese stick	Apple and granola bar	Apple and nuts	Apple and nuts	Apple and nuts	X	X
Snack #2	Greek yogurt and berries	Carrots and hummus	Greek yogurt and berries	Carrots and hummus	Carrots and hummus	X	X

Planning Your Meals: Put It on Paper

Now it's your turn. Write these charts on a piece of paper. You are also welcome to combine them to reflect your general eating pattern if that makes it easier to visualize. Side note: I used meal #1, #2, #3 because it's okay to eat whatever you want at these meals. You don't have to eat breakfast foods for breakfast. I have also identified the seven days of the week by their names, but remember, flexibility over rigid meal planning is key for ADHDers. You can eat your Friday meal on Monday. It's okay.

Meal	Mon	Tues	Wed	Thurs	Fri	Sat	Sun
Meal #1							
Meal #2							
Meal #3							

Snack	Mon	Tues	Wed	Thurs	Fri	Sat	Sun
Snack #1							
Snack #2							

Next, follow these steps:

1. Cross off any days, meals, or snacks that you don't need to plan for, including meals you eat out or get delivery.

2. Do you have any meals or snacks that are automated like my breakfast? If so, fill them in.

3. How many meals do you feel comfortable cooking each week. Two? Three? Fill in when you think you will cook them (remember it's okay if that changes).

4. How many servings of leftovers will you have? If you make one extra portion for each meal and make three meals, you will have leftovers for three meals. If you make two extra portions for each meal, you will have leftovers for six meals. Fill these in.

5. Do you have any blank spots? Fill in any blank meals or snacks with something you know you will eat. For example, if I had a blank snack, I'd add one of my go-to snacks like carrots and hummus. It's 100 percent okay if this changes. The goal of this is to make sure that you plan enough meals.

Meal Planning Tools and Strategies for ADHDers

Now that we've discussed the basics of meal planning, let's talk about some specific strategies and options for making this easier for the ADHD brain.

Day-of Meal Planning

Our first strategy is Day-of Meal Planning. This is exactly what it sounds like: deciding what to eat on the day you plan to eat it. This strategy is great if you struggle with planning too far in advance. If this is you, I recommend using this strategy only for dinners and automating snacks, breakfast, and lunch. You may be able to do this with other meals if you work from home, you're a stay-at-home parent, or retired. This strategy does require some work up front to learn what food items you frequently use (vegetable broth, canned beans, frozen chicken, etc.) so you can stock your pantry and refrigerator with those items. You also need to have the financial resources to keep a well-stocked pantry, have extra freezer space, the cooking skills to get creative with what you have on hand, and a more flexible schedule to go to the grocery store more often if needed.

If you can stock your freezer with protein, veggies, etc. and your pantry with cooking essentials that you or your family commonly use, then you could avoid having to plan for the week. With Day-of Meal Planning, you will likely need to do one grocery trip a week to restock on basics and pick up a few fresh items based on what's on sale that week like meat, vegetables, etc.

"Pick Three" Meal Planning

This is a favorite strategy of mine because it is so flexible. It involves picking three meals to make for the week. You can do this for all three daily meals or just dinners. If you do this for dinners, then plan to make enough to have leftovers for one or two additional meals. So these three meals would cover six to nine meals that week depending on how many additional servings you make. The leftovers can be eaten the next day for lunch or dinner another night of the week. I combine this strategy with another strategy—delivery meal kits—to make meal planning work really well for me.

Automating Meals

Automating some of your meals may not sound intuitive to some folks. But most of us can't just decide in the moment what we want to eat and then go make it for all of our meals and snacks. Automating some of your eating can be extremely helpful if deciding what to eat feels like a full-time job.

Think of it as creating a predetermined option or options for eating that makes it easier to implement/initiate the task of making food and eating it. It takes some of the guesswork out of deciding what to eat, helps you identify if you need to pick up an ingredient, and if you need to delegate or ask for help. When you know your sensory preferences, you can make sure the meals and snacks that you automate fulfill those preferences so you still have enjoyable eating experiences.

Examples of automating meals include:

- Having a predetermined daily snack, like apple slices with almond butter
- Planning to have a frozen meal for dinner on Thursdays because you know you never have the energy to make a meal that night
- Having two options for a ready-to-go breakfast, like a protein drink and a banana or overnight oats, because you are too tired to make decisions in the morning.

Use AI

AI is a great tool to help with meal planning. It's a way to automate some of the decision-making. You can ask it to plan out your meals, taking into account the foods you want or need to use before they go bad, your sensory preferences, dietary preferences, and how much time you want to spend on meals. Ask it to select meals, make a grocery list, and include directions for you. You will likely need to tweak the results, but it will give you a good starting point.

Theme Nights

This is another strategy to automate meal planning. It gives you a framework to work within. Instead of a million options, you know you're having some version of tacos on Tuesday. It gives you some predictability, but also leaves room for variety and novelty. This strategy can be great for feeding a family. Your kids will know what to expect for dinner. You could do this for every night of the week or have a couple theme nights.

Examples of theme nights include:

- Meatless Monday (plant-based meals)
- Mediterranean Monday
- Taco Tuesday
- Wrap Wednesday
- Thai Food Tuesday
- Fish Friday or Seafood Sunday
- Spaghetti (pasta) Saturday
- Soup and Salad Sunday
- Breakfast for Dinner Night
- Lunch for Dinner Night (think sandwiches)
- Stir-Fry Night
- Pasta Night
- Mediterranean Night
- Pizza Night
- Crockpot/InstantPot Night
- Clean-Out-the-Fridge Night

Meal Kit Services

I am a big fan of meal kit services for ADHDers. They are extremely helpful during busy seasons of life.

The pros of meal kits include:

- You can learn how to cook or learn different cooking techniques
- You can try new cuisines without having to commit to ALL the spices, herbs, and specialty ingredients
- Makes grocery shopping easier because you don't have to buy as much at the store
- Limits choices with meal planning
- Decreases food waste
- May save money, especially if you eat out a lot
- May have visual directions or come with recipe cards

The cons of meal kits include:

- May cost more per meal if you cook at home
- Hard if you have a big family
- May not accommodate your dietary needs
- Still may need to purchase basics/essentials
- The meals might feel repetitive over time

There are many different kinds of meal kit services, so you can pick which works best for you and your life. If you're considering trying one, here are a few tips on how to pick recipes:

- Choose recipes with a suggested cooking times that are under 30 minutes.
- Look for methods that use fewer utensils and steps to reduce how much you have to prep before cooking and clean up after. One-pot or one-pan meals are your friend!
- Any recipe labelled "no chopping" is also your friend.
- Are any of your favorites on the menu for the week? Save them so you can remember them for the future!
- When you're choosing a recipe, review it first to make sure you have all the tools you need and you know how to perform all the instructions listed.
- Try to aim for meals with different proteins, veggies, and carbs so you get a variety of nutrients across the week.

Create a Nutrition 9-1-1 Plan

This one is less of a strategy for successful meal planning and more a strategy for what to do when meal planning fails (which happens sometimes, and that's okay!). A nutrition 9-1-1 plan is an emergency plan—basically, a reference list—of your go-to meals and snacks.

These should be low spoon options that you can make when you're exhausted, forgot to create a meal plan, are short on time, have limited options on hand, or don't have an appetite, but know you need to eat something. It doesn't have to be a set list; you can always add new meals and snacks as your tastes evolve and you get more comfortable in the kitchen.

To create your nutrition 9-1-1 plan:

1. Get out a piece of paper and something to write with.
2. Set a timer for no more than 30 minutes.
3. Make a list of your go-tos for breakfast, lunch, dinner, and snacks. Include frozen meals.
4. Next to each meal write how many spoons it requires.
5. Make a list of meals you frequently eat order or eat out.

Whatever meal planning tools or system you develop, remember to keep it simple so you'll be able to use it during a busy week or when you don't have a lot of spoons. Find ways to be flexible so you can make adjustments to work with your ADHD brain instead of against it. Remember that automation is your friend and can help you save some spoons in the meal planning process. And always have a plan B or nutrition 9-1-1 plan to fall back on, because things often don't go as planned.

Next, we are going to tackle grocery shopping so you can get the items you need to execute your meal plan.

Grocery Shopping

After you've made your plan, it's time to gather your ingredients. This likely means you will need to go grocery shopping or place an order for pick-up or delivery. Grocery stores can be a sensory hell for some ADHDers. The awful fluorescent lighting, loud music, people, lines, and all the options combine to create the perfect storm for sensory overload. Not to mention the difficulty of trying to find everything on your list, while also trying to avoid making a bunch of impulse purchases. But don't despair! The tools and strategies in this section can go a long way toward making grocery shopping if not pleasant, than at least less painful, for the ADHD brain.

The Basics: How to Create a Shopping List

If you're new to grocery list making, I recommend grouping items by category. Search Google for grocery list templates several options will pop up. Or, you can freestyle it. If you are starting from scratch, here few suggestions:

1. First fill in your essentials. Are there items that you need to restock? My essentials include: avocados, apples, carrots, peppers, cucumber, eggs, milk, bread, a snack item, a frozen meal, snacking cheese, some kind of dip.

2. Review your meal plan. Cross off the items you already have for those meals. Add the items you need to buy to your list.

3. Visualize. It can be helpful to place items on the list in an order that's similar to where they can be found in the store. I know my stores really well, so I am able to visualize walking through the store and adding the items I need from each section to my list.

Before you walk out the door to leave for the store, think "phone, keys, wallet/purse, **list**, reusable bags." You might forget the list. I forget my list A LOT, but writing it out helps me to remember it, so I make it part of my meal planning process. Determine if you prefer a paper or a digital list. Digital lists can be made using an app, the notes feature on your phone, or you can even text it to yourself or your partner.

Personally, I will get distracted if I take my phone out at the store, so a paper list works better for me. When I write a list and forget it, I either ask my partner to send me a picture of the list or try to shop from memory. If I try to do it from memory, I always do an extra lap or two around the store before checking out, because I will likely find a couple of things I forgot from the list.

CSA Boxes

While not meal kits, per se, Community Supported Agriculture (CSA) boxes can be a great option for getting fresh produce and/or meat every week. This may be a good fit for you if you like to use your own recipes but want to take the hassle out of choosing and sourcing ingredients every week. These can come with produce you may have never heard of before, so it can require a little extra work in terms of figuring out how to cook or use them.

Grocery Shopping Tools and Strategies for ADHDers

Now that we've discussed the basics of grocery list making, let's talk about some specific strategies and options for making shopping for groceries easier for the ADHD brain.

Avoid Peak Hours

I know this may not be an option for everyone. If you find grocery shopping overwhelming but don't want to outsource grocery shopping for pick up or delivery, it might be helpful to shop when the grocery store is less busy. I try to avoid shopping from 10:00 am to 5:00 pm on the weekends at all costs.

Check Google Maps for the peak hours and avoid shopping during those times. If you have no choice, at least you can be mentally prepared for the crowds. If you need to shop on the weekends, early morning or after dinner are probably going to be the best times to go.

Shop Sensory-Friendly Hours

In November 2023, Walmart rolled out sensory-friendly hours nationwide to create a better shopping environment for neurodiverse individuals. In the United States, all Walmart stores offer sensory-friendly hours from 8:00 am to 10:00 am, seven days a week. They dim their obnoxiously bright lights, turn off the music, and turn the TVs to a static image. Let's hope that by the time you're reading this book there will be more stores offering special hours or even making permanent, more sensory-friendly changes to their spaces.

Pick a Primary Grocery Store

If you live somewhere with multiple grocery stores nearby, you might want to pick one of them as your primary store. This can help you learn the store layout, find out when they typically restock, and become familiar with some of the employees. Going to the same store regularly can also help you get used to the parking lot, lighting, sounds, smells, etc.

Outsource: Order for Pickup or Delivery

If you find grocery shopping takes up too many spoons, consider outsourcing it. You can order groceries online for pickup or delivery. And pickup is generally free! If you like, you can save outsourcing for certain situations, such as busy or stressful weeks when you know you could use those spoons for something else. Or you can reserve outsourcing for items you forgot, to restock your essentials, or when you're out of town and it would be helpful to have groceries waiting for you when you return.

The pros of ordering groceries include:

- Easy to reorder
- May decrease impulse shopping
- Saves you time and energy
- Allows you to delegate shopping to someone else
- Removes chances of forgetting items

The cons of ordering groceries include:

- The ADHD tax: membership fees, delivery fees, higher prices than in-store, tipping shoppers
- You cannot hand-select items like fruits, vegetables, deli meats or seafood items, etc.
- Unpredictable shopper/selection
- May miss new items at the store
- Lack of novelty

Try Smaller Grocery Stores

If I do go to the grocery store, I like to shop at smaller grocery stores such as Trader Joe's or ALDI. It's true that sometimes the selection at smaller grocery stores can be unpredictable. They don't have everything. Over time, you'll remember what items they don't carry. If you have very specific preferences for certain brands, you may not find them at these stores.

On the other hand, these stores can be way less overwhelming because of their smaller layout and fewer choices. Trying to decide between twenty different types of pasta sauces is hard when you are indecisive. Prices are oftentimes better at the smaller stores. And, here's a bonus! They have more seasonal items, which means there's novelty.

Buying in Bulk

Costco or Sam's Club are great options to buy in bulk. You may want to buy in bulk if you want to save money, decrease the frequency of your shopping, or if you have a family you need to feed. An extra freezer might be worth the investment if you like to buy in bulk or batch cook and freeze.

Items to consider buying in bulk include:

- Meat, poultry, fish (extra freezer space may be required)
- Starches you use frequently, such as rice, quinoa, or oatmeal
- Olive oil, cooking spray
- Herbs and spices you use often (salt, pepper, garlic powder, cinnamon, etc.)
- Snacks
- Frozen items
- Cleaning products
- Paper products

Consider Asking for Support

My partner and I love grocery shopping together. It's a way for us to spend some quality time together. We try to hold each other accountable for sticking to our list and find it helpful to have an extra set of eyes so we don't forget anything. We might divide up some of the list.

If you live alone, you could ask a friend to be your grocery shopping buddy. This could help establish a day and time that you regularly shop. Having someone you know with you can make the shopping experience feel more comfortable.

Use ADHD-Friendly Tools

Noise-canceling headphones are a great tool for ADHDers who struggle with sensory overwhelm in the grocery store. They decrease sensory input to limit distractions and sensory overwhelm. There are also some really excellent earplug brands now that can help reduce some of the noise. I usually just use my AirPods.

Hopefully, you discovered some new strategies to help make grocery shopping easier for you. Let's move on to the next step in making food: Kitchen Organization.

Getting Your Kitchen Organized

As an ADHDer, I have learned that if a task feels harder or more unmanageable than it should be, one of the first things I should do first is evaluate my environment. Take the kitchen. A messy, unorganized kitchen is going to make it harder for you to make food. This is because it's creating more tasks that you have to complete (washing dishes, clearing the counter, wiping down the stove) before you can even begin to make food.

A clean, well-organized kitchen makes it easier to initiate the task of cooking. Consider the flow of your cooking space. Are there any adjustments you could make to make it easier to get started or decrease the friction between the steps in the process?

The goal is to remove things that get in the way of cooking. These can be really small changes that make a big difference, such as moving utensils, ingredients, and recipes closer to the stove to make them more accessible. When these things are hard to find or grab, just gathering what you need can become a big task in your ADHD brain.

Having a well-organized kitchen can also help reduce food waste and overbuying, because it's easier to remember, find, and use the food you already have.

To be clear, your kitchen doesn't need to look as if it was featured on an episode of Marie Kondo's show. It just needs be ordered in a way that works for your brain.

A few general tips include:

- Give yourself permission to make your kitchen work for you and your brain, even if that means it's not perfect aesthetically. Don't get caught in the trap of comparing your kitchen to some influencer's on social media. If you need to label things, do it! If you need open cabinets so you see things and use them, do it!
- You can change where things live. If you find yourself always opening a drawer for silverware and the silverware is in a different drawer, then switch the drawers!
- We'll talk about this more later but, keep in mind that cleaning is morally neutral. Your moral worth is not determined by how clean your kitchen or house is. When you make cleaning morally neutral it takes some of the shame out of struggling to keep up with it.

Kitchen Organization Tools and Strategies for ADHDers

Before we start discussing organization tools and strategies, I want to note that there are entire books dedicated to this topic. We're going to discuss some quick tips and tools to get your started in this area. If this is something you want to learn more about, I highly recommend checking out resources from other ADHD professionals that specialize in organizing your kitchen and living space.

Use Tools

Invest in organization tools, gadgets, and appliances that solve a problem you regularly experience or reduce the barrier to doing something you struggle with. To make it easier to wash and dry dishes, find a drying rack that works for you. Clear airtight food storage containers for dry goods, fruits, veggies, and other food items not only reduce visual clutter, but allow you to easily identify what's inside. A label maker and labels can make it easier to remember what goes where. Keep your cabinets more organized with racks for pots, lids, and storage containers.

I would consider these tools an ADHD tax. They may not be a necessity for a lot of people, but they will make your kitchen more functional and organized, so don't hesitate to use them if you need them.

Pantry Organization Tips

Store similar items together such as canned goods, dry starches, or breakfast foods. Another way to organize is to group items that are regularly used together. For example, you could have a bin for overnight oats ingredients so you can easily access everything you need quickly at the end of a long day.

You may want to use clear bins to store similar items together. This makes it easy to see everything at a glance. Some potential dry food storage groupings are:

- Canned Goods: beans, soups, vegetables, broths
- Dry Starches: rice, quinoa, pasta, etc.
- Breakfast Foods: cereals, oatmeal, granola
- Grab and Go Snacks: granola bars, nuts, chips
- Kids Snacks
- Baking Supplies: flour, sugar, chocolate chips

Refrigerator and Freezer Organization Tips

Don't put produce in the crisper drawer. That's where produce goes to die. Store it in airtight containers in the door or at eye level on a shelf so you see it. (See next section for more tips for fruits and veggies.) Instead use the crisper drawers for beverages, sauces, salad dressings, and other condiments.

The freezer is your friend, especially if food goes bad in your fridge. If you have the space, consider getting a standalone freezer. This allows you to buy meats and other frozen foods you use in bulk to save money. Freeze bread so it doesn't mold. You can also freeze veggie scraps and veggies that may be starting to go bad to use in a flavorful homemade vegetable broth.

Below are two tables that show how to store fruits and veggies so that they last longer. If you don't have the spoons to store things this way that is okay. But if you find that your produce keeps going bad it might be helpful to explore some of these strategies.

Vegetable	Storage	How Long It Can Last
Asparagus, celery, carrots	Fridge in jar with water, cover with plastic bag	2–3 weeks
Brussel Sprouts	Fridge in plastic bag	3–5 weeks
Broccoli	Fridge in damp paper towel	10–14 days
Dark leafy greens & salad greens	Plastic bag with paper towel	10–14 days 2–3 weeks
Cauliflower	Fridge in plastic bag	2–4 weeks
Cucumber	Fridge wrapped in plastic or bees wrap	10–14 days
Zucchini & summer squash	Room temp in ventilated plastic bag	2 weeks
Onion	Dark, cool, dry area	4–6 weeks
Tomatoes	Room temp & out of direct sunlight	1–3 weeks
Peppers	Unwashed in a plastic bag	2–3 weeks
Garlic	Fridge, dry, dark, ventilated areas	6–7 months

Fruit	Storage	How Long It Can Last
Apples	Fridge, ventilated bags	1–12 months
Berries	Fridge, unwashed with paper towel	5–7 days
Avocado	Room temp. If ripe, in fridge.	varies
Grapes	Fridge, airtight container	2–3 weeks
Citrus	Shelf in fridge	2–3 weeks
Cherries	Fridge, wrapped in plastic bag	2–3 weeks
Stonefruit	Counter until ripe, then move to fridge	2–5 weeks

Fruit and Veggie Storage Tips

As previously stated, I recommend storing produce in airtight containers in your fridge door or at eye level so you will see them and use them. If you don't use airtight containers, they will spoil faster. Keep fridge below 40°F (4°C) to slow bacteria growth, and separate ethylene gas producers from produce that is sensitive to ethylene gas. This gas will cause produce to ripen faster.

Ethylene gas producers	Sensitive to ethylene gas
Apples, bananas, kiwis, nectarines, peaches, plums, apricots, avocados, honeydew, mangoes, papayas, pears, tomatoes	Broccoli, carrots, eggplants, lettuce, potatoes, asparagus, cucumbers, green beans, cauliflower, watermelon

Hire a Professional Organizer

If organizing your kitchen takes too many spoons, consider hiring a professional organizer to help you. Organization is an executive function that you might struggle with, so if you have the means to outsource it, don't hesitate.

ADHDers can thrive with the right systems. Getting an expert to help with organizing can save you time and energy. Objective opinions can be helpful when you struggle with figuring out whether or not you really need to keep things. But make sure that you're hiring the right organizer, preferably one with experience working with ADHD clients. Here are a few questions to ask before hiring:

- What kinds of projects do you specialize in?
- Have you completed any training or certifications?
- What is your typical approach? Do you give homework?
- Have you ever worked with anyone who has ADHD or is neurodivergent? How did you tailor your approach to accommodate their needs?
- Do you offer a contract or other written agreement?
- Can you provide a portfolio or references?

So far, you've planned your meals, bought your ingredients, and organized them in your kitchen in a way that works for you. Next step: food prep.

Food Prep

Food preparation includes all the steps leading up to cooking food. This includes gathering ingredients, thawing them, chopping and cutting, measuring them, marinating or seasoning, organizing equipment, preheating appliances, and more.

There's A LOT that goes into prep, which is why it can be a challenge for ADHDers. The goal of simplifying food preparation is to save you time and energy and decrease overwhelm. Like everything else you might struggle with consistently doing these things, but learning to implement them more often can make cooking easier.

Common barriers to food prep for ADHDers include:

- Remembering to do all of the steps
- Chopping and cutting feel tedious
- Time blindness
- Staying organized
- Not getting distracted

Food Prep Strategies for ADHDers

At some point, someone's probably asked you if you've tried spending a few hours on Sunday meal prepping. And you probably answered, "Yes, and that doesn't work for me."

If this method does work for you, that's great. But if not, it might make you feel like a failure. You're not a failure, you're just trying to do something that may not work with your ADHD brain. So what are some alternatives when it comes to food prep?

Don't Eat the Frog, Eat the Ice Cream

I learned this trick from Jesse Anderson, author of *Extra Focus: The Quick Start Guide to Adult ADHD*. "Eat the frog" is a common strategy for procrastination where you do the most difficult task first. For ADHD brains it's not about how

difficult a task is, but how much energy it might use, so "Eat the frog" often doesn't work for our brains. Meal prep can use up a lot of energy. So instead of eating the frog, eat the ice cream—start with a task that excites you or one that is easy to do and gives you a small win. This will provide the momentum to do more difficult tasks. An example of this for me is going to Trader Joe's (the fun task) and coming home and batch cooking chicken for the week (the more difficult task).

Selective Meal Prep

Instead of prepping full meals, consider only prepping the parts of a meal or snack. Pick the parts you struggle with the most with or do the tasks that will make the job easier later. Two common examples from my clients are washing and cutting up fruit or veggies in advance and batch cooking proteins. Completing both of these tasks ahead of time will make it easier to cook food throughout the week. Some ADHDers find that if they outsource shopping, it means they have the spoons to do advance food prep when their groceries arrive.

Read the Recipe at Least Two Times—and Do It Early

Do I remember to do this every time? Nope. Do I regret it when I'm trying a new recipe and three steps in the directions say to quickly add something that I don't have ready so I end up burning the food? Every time. Read the recipe before you start cooking. I know it's annoying, but if you have a general idea of the steps, making the recipe won't be as chaotic as if you are learning as you go along.

If I'm making a new recipe for dinner, I usually read it earlier in the day so my brain has an idea of what the process will be. This makes it easier to get started. Then, I like to read the recipe out loud right before I start cooking. I also prefer to work from a paper copy of the recipe so I don't get distracted on my phone.

Mise en Place

Have you ever noticed on cooking shows how they have all the ingredients and utensils set out and ready to go? That is mise en place. It's chopping the veggies, measuring out spices, etc., *before you start cooking*. It makes ingredients more accessible and cooking a smoother process. Sometimes I like to imagine I'm on a cooking show to make it easier to do this.

Use Shortcuts for Fruits and Veggies

Fresh fruits and vegetables will likely need to be cleaned, cut, chopped, minced, etc. For a lot of ADHDers, this takes too many spoons. Make it easier on yourself by using shortcuts such as:

- Wash, prep, and store fruits and veggies as soon as you bring them home. If you order groceries, then you might find you actually have the energy to do this step.

- Prep all your veggies when you cook instead of just prepping the veggies you need for that meal.
- Use frozen produce. This saves you the steps of washing the produce, taking out a cutting board and knife, and cleaning up. Frozen fruits and veggies are just as nutritious as fresh and often less expensive.
- Invest in a veggie chopper/mandolin. I've heard from many ADHDers that this makes it easier to cut fresh produce.
- Buy pre-cut fruit, veggies and meats. Yes, there is an ADHD tax with these. They are probably still less money than buying produce and having it rot in your fridge and then needing to buy more or order takeout instead. You may not always need to buy pre-cut, but you can use them as needed to help make cooking more accessible.

Now that we've got everything prepped, let's move on to the most important step: cooking.

Cooking

Cooking is a skill that takes time, repetition, and patience to develop. That being said, you don't have to be a professional chef to make tasty food. You may not know how to cook and that is okay. But if you want to eat more meals at home, it can be helpful to learn some basic cooking skills.

Lack of experience is often one of the biggest barriers to cooking (this goes for anyone, but especially for ADHDers). If this is you, there are lots of resources to help you learn. If you learn by watching others, then search for cooking

demonstrations on YouTube or watch cooking shows. You can also ask a family member, friend, or partner if you can watch them while they cook. I learned so much from my parents by simply spending time with them in the kitchen while they cooked. As I got older, I got more involved.

If you learn better by doing, you could ask someone to teach you how to make their favorite recipe, invest in cooking classes, or experiment on your own.

Cooking Strategies for ADHDers

Aside from lack of experience, barriers to cooking for ADHDers include the usual suspects: time, organization, overwhelm, task initiation, and low energy. Let's talk strategies for how to overcome these common challenges and get to cooking!

Invest in ADHD-Friendly Kitchen Appliances

There are tons of kitchen gadgets on the market, but a lot of them you just don't need. You don't need every tool listed here either, but investing in a few of them could end up saving you a ton of time and energy. Here are my best recommendations.

- **Air fryer.** If I could pick one kitchen appliance to have forever, it would be an air fryer. You can cook food from frozen, you don't have to wait for your oven to preheat, and it takes much less time.
- **InstantPot/pressure cooker/slow cooker.** These are great if you like to batch cook or do dump and cook meals like chilis, soups, etc.
- **Rice cooker.** This can save you some headspace when cooking. You just dump the water, rice, and any necessary seasonings into the machine and press a button to cook it. You don't have to pay attention to the cook time or worry about burning it.
- **Blender with cup attachments.** A good blender is worth the investment if you like smoothies. Buying a blender with cup attachments can save you a step in the clean-up process.

Aside from these gadgets, I also recommend buying multiples of kitchen utensils that you use often like spatulas, measuring spoons and cups, cutting boards, pans, etc. You might have more dishes to do eventually, but it can help decrease how often you need to do your dishes or make it possible to cook when you haven't done the dishes.

Music

Music makes everything more enjoyable in my opinion. You could make a playlist for cooking. I love listening to old music like Frank Sinatra when I cook. It romanticizes the process of cooking for me and it's not overly distracting. Having music on means I'm more relaxed and probably dancing while I cook.

Use the Power of Connection

Find ways to get others involved. If you live alone call a friend while you cook. Even better, call a friend to body double and cook together. You can invite family or friends over if you enjoy cooking for others. During the pandemic my best friend and I would take turns cooking a meal for each other (she left NYC to stay with me right before lockdown started so we were in a COVID bubble together). Ask your partner, roommate, or kids to sit with you while you cook or ask them to help in some way.

Tap into Your Creative Side

Use cooking as an opportunity to tap into your creative side. ADHDers are creative people and problem solvers. These skills can be valuable in the kitchen and may even explain why some ADHDers make fantastic chefs. The more comfortable you get in the kitchen the easier it will be to put your own spin on a recipe or come up with a recipe using random ingredients in your pantry.

Cleanup

An icebreaker question I ask my clients in my small group coaching program is "would you rather have someone wash your dishes or do your laundry?" Both of these tasks are chores that ADHDers often loathe and avoid until their sink is overflowing or they're down to their last pair of clean underwear. I'm not going to discuss strategies for keeping up with your laundry here, but we are going to talk about the dishes and some of these strategies may transfer!

Your kitchen doesn't have to be spotless. The state of your kitchen says nothing about the type of person you are. You might be better at cleaning if you enjoy it or if you also have OCD. But cleaning is a monotonous task that pretty much never ends. Even when I think I'm done doing the dishes, I somehow find a cup in plain sight.

> If cleaning is an area of life you struggle with, I highly recommend the book *How to Keep House While Drowning* by KC Davis. She encourages you to think of cleaning as a morally neutral care task. In other words, you are not a failure because you can't keep up with the dishes.

Kitchen Cleanup Tools and Strategies for ADHDers

Barriers to cleaning the kitchen for ADHDers include sensory overload, lack of a system or routine, lack of time, and boredom. Let's go over some strategies for helping with these.

Determine Your Bare Minimum

Instead of trying to meet neurotypical cleaning standards, determine what your nonnegotiables are for cleaning or tidying your kitchen space after a meal. What is the bare minimum you can realistically commit to keeping up with on a daily basis (or whatever frequency feels realistic for you)? I recommend tidying on a daily basis because I've found that starting the day with a messy kitchen or living space means you're starting the day with more overwhelm and distractions. It only gets worse as the day goes on.

My bare minimum includes:

- Wiping down counters at the end of the day
- Rinse all bowls, plates, silverware, cups, pots and pans and place in sink
- Put away leftovers
- Put items back in their homes

Your bare minimum might look different than this. That's okay. Do whatever works for you. And if you're struggling with this, ask yourself, how would your future self feel to wake up to a clean, or at least cleaner, kitchen?

Setting Realistic Expectations

It's really easy to create expectations based on neurotypical standards or to set your expectations too high if you have perfectionistic tendencies. Setting realistic expectations around cleaning means asking yourself what you can realistically do without taking up too much time or making it feeling like too much

I recommend establishing your personal baseline for your space and deciding how often you can reset that space back to baseline. For me, I try to get my kitchen back to baseline or do a reset at least once a week. Some weeks I can get my kitchen back to baseline daily, but other weeks it piles up.

Reset Day

Pick a day of the week when you will spend a specified amount of time getting your kitchen back to baseline. Write a list of the major tasks you want done and then break each task down into smaller tasks. Breaking down tasks can make them feel more doable and give you actionable steps. If you are unsure of how to break down tasks, try using an AI tool. It might not get it perfect, but it can give you a list to adjust to your needs.

Body Double

I have no problem doing the dishes when I have someone to talk to. So, I often do the dishes while FaceTiming my ADHD bestie or talking to my sister on the phone. If your kids sit and do homework in the kitchen, do the dishes then. FaceTime a friend (they probably also need to be neurodivergent) or join a virtual body doubling group.

Delegate

Asking for help can be hard as an ADHDer. You might be afraid of being rejected or feel like you shouldn't need help with cleaning. But there is no shame in asking for the help you need.

Unless it's been agreed upon, no one in the household should be responsible for doing all the meal planning, grocery shopping, cooking, and cleaning. It places an unnecessary burden on one person in the house, which is extremely unfair. If you've never discussed responsibilities around food with your partner or family, you might want to. It might be an uncomfortable conversation.

If you have a partner, you're a team. Play off of each other's strengths. Is one of you better at cooking? Is one of you better at cleaning? Can you divide up parts of cooking? For example, in college my then-boyfriend would cook the protein part of the meal and I would prepare the vegetables or salad.

If one person cooks, the other cleans. If someone does the cooking and cleaning, the other should be doing the shopping or prepping, or other boring household tasks.

Develop a System for the Dishes

Keeping up with dishes can big a big barrier to cooking for some ADHDers. If that's you, you're not alone! But there are a lot of different ways you can approach dishes to make them easier. Get curious and figure out what works for you. Here are a few examples of systems to make doing the dishes easier:

- **Clean as you go.** While something is simmering on the stove, baking in the oven, on the grill, etc., try to clean up. Filling your sink with soapy, warm water can make this easier. When you're done using a kitchen tool you can toss it in the sink to soak. (I would probably avoid putting knives directly in the sink to avoid forgetting and potentially cutting yourself.)
- **Do dishes at the same time every day.** Most of the time, I do not do my dishes every time after I eat. I typically rinse my dishes and leave them in the sink until the end of the day, when I load and run my dishwasher. I empty it in the morning. On low energy weeks or weeks when my spoons are used up in other places, the dishes pile up for a few days until I get to them.
- **Organize the sink.** If you fill your sink with dishes before emptying it to wash them, try to organize how dishes and utensils go into it. This helps remove some visual chaos and can help streamline the process when you finally do your dishes. After you rinse something off, sort and stack similar items together: plates with other plates, bowls with other bowls, etc.
- **Just do one.** To overcome a sink full of dirty dishes, try the "just do one" approach. This strategy can help with task initiation. Can you put one dish in the dishwasher? You only have to do one of whatever it is you're trying to get started with doing. That's enough. But doing one shows your brain that you can do it and your brain might decide it can do more.

Have the Right Tools to Make Cleanup Easier

The right tools can make all the difference. These tools can help accommodate your sensory needs. This can decrease overwhelm and help make it easier to keep up with the dishes. Here are a few that I recommend:

RUBBER GLOVES

Washing dishes can be a sensory-ick. Wearing gloves means you don't actually have to touch all that leftover, half-eaten food. It can help you stay on task and serves as a cue for your brain to associate that when you wear these gloves it means it's time to do the dishes. It can also prevent dry skin on your hands and keep your fingers from getting pruney.

APRON

One day I will have higher counters so I don't get splashed with water. You could use an apron for cooking and doing the dishes. Just like the rubber gloves, an apron can be a cue to remind your brain of the task you're about to do.

ANTI-FATIGUE MATS

Anti-fatigue mats can create a more comfortable environment, especially if you find it challenging to stand in the kitchen while you cook or clean.

THE RIGHT DISH SOAP

If you have hyposensitivities to smells, you might want to find a dish soap that has a scent you really like. This can make it a more enjoyable sensory experience. On the other hand, if you are hypersensitive to smells, you might want to select a fragrance-free or mildly scented dish soap. If you wash your dishes without gloves you might want a moisturizing dish soap.

VISUAL TIMER

Visual timers are a great tool for ADHDers. You can use a timer to learn how long it actually takes you to do tasks. Boring tasks can feel like they take forever to complete so you put them off. Only to realize that a task only takes 15 minutes to do once you finally do it. Write down how long it takes you to do specific cleaning tasks. Keep a list of these tasks and times somewhere visible in your kitchen space so you can remind your brain that it actually takes 15 minutes to load the dishwasher, not forever like your brain might tell you.

MUSIC

Music does wonders when you're cooking or cleaning up. Music allows me to have fun while I'm cleaning. I sing along and break out some of my awesomely awkward dance moves while I clean. Podcasts and audiobooks are also a great option.

HEADPHONES OR NOISE-CANCELLING HEADPHONES

These can also be a cue. Reduce sensory input to reduce overwhelm.

It's Okay If You Struggle with Cleaning

Struggling with cleaning can bring a lot of shame. If you've struggled with this since childhood, you probably hear nagging voices like, "You're such a slob" "It takes no extra time to put your dish in the dishwasher" or "It's not that hard to wash your dishes after you eat" from parents, roommates, etc. But you are not lazy, a slob, careless, or anything else. You have ADHD and struggle with executive function.

Cleaning is a boring task that NEVER ends. Don't get me wrong I love a clean kitchen, but as an ADHDer it's not easy to keep up with cleaning. If cleaning is something that requires a lot of spoons, consider delegating it by hiring a cleaner. Yes, this is an ADHD tax and requires some financial privilege.

This might require challenging some internalized ableism because you might feel like you "should" be able to clean your living space on your own. There is nothing wrong with asking for help in areas of your life that you struggle with, especially if these are things that drain you. It's okay to save your spoons to do other things that bring you joy, social connection, etc.

Now, that you've learned some strategies for simplifying all the steps in the process of feeding yourself, it's finally time to make some food. In chapter 9 I will share some simple and fast recipes to show you how to put the tips from these last two chapters into practice!

Your Kids Involved

If you have kids, you can 100 percent delegate doing parts of the cleaning process to them based on their age. Maybe it's not all the dishes. Maybe they do the plates, silverware, cups, and bowls, and you do the pots and pans/big stuff. Here's a brief list of age-appropriate kitchen-related chores:

- Ages 2-3: put away groceries
- Ages 4-5: remove plates from table
- Ages 6-7: wipe kitchen counters, load and start dishwasher (parents sort), assist with cooking simple foods
- Ages 7-9: load and unload dishwasher, help with meal prep, pack own lunch
- Ages 10+ prepare a simple meal

CHAPTER 9

Easy Non-Diet Recipes for Adults with ADHD

The recipes in this chapter are recipes that my clients and I find ADHD-friendly. What makes them ADHD-friendly? They use minimal ingredients, incorporate shortcut foods, don't take longer than 45 minutes (most take significantly less), and use minimal utensils for easier clean up. These recipes also incorporate the principles of gentle nutrition.

The chapter is divided into six sections. Breakfasts and Smoothies is for ADHDers who don't mind cooking breakfast (though smoothies can technically be consumed at any time of the day). No-Heat and Handheld Meals are great to bring on the go for school or work. One-Pot and One-Pan Meals has great options if washing dishes is a barrier to cooking for you. And then there's the Air Fryer Meals section. I really do think this gadget is worth the hype for ADHDers. With an air fryer you don't have to remember to preheat the oven, foods cook much faster, and you can cook straight from frozen, which is great if you forget to thaw food in advance. The Veggie-Focused Recipes section is for my vegetarian or vegan ADHDers, while Fancy Classics are for all the ADHDers who have a child's flavor palette or enjoy "kid foods," but want to find ways to ADD ingredients to make more nutrient-dense meals. Finally, I am a huge fan of convenience snacks, so I included some sweet and savory options in the final section of the chapter.

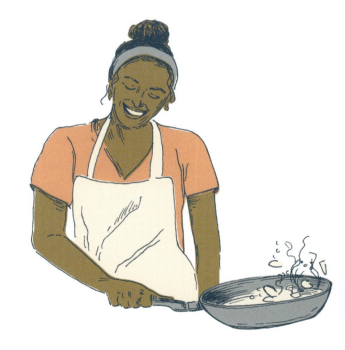

I hope you find these recipes useful and delicious and feel empowered to start experimenting in the kitchen. Enjoy!

Overnight Oats

There are so many benefits to consuming oats, but I don't recommend eating them on their own. When I eat oats, whether hot or cold, I treat them as a base carbohydrate that needs to be "dressed up" with some extra protein, fat, and fiber to make a filling meal. The following overnight oats recipes do just that with three delicious options for making a satisfying breakfast.

Overnight oats are typically eaten cold, but you can microwave them if you prefer warm oatmeal. If you make these a lot, consider storing the ingredients you use most in one bin so you can just pull it out instead of gathering everything from different parts of the pantry.

Overnight oats may be a breakfast worth "prepping" because you can make a week's worth of meals at once. If you do this, multiply the recipe ingredients by the number of meals you want to make. You can find overnight oats in the grocery store as well. If you go this route, keep in mind that you may want to add more toppings. The serving sizes are not usually enough for breakfast in my opinion.

Yield: 1 serving

Ingredients

Overnight Oats Base
- ½ cup (40 g) old fashioned oats
- ½ cup (118 ml) milk of choice
- ¼ cup (65 g) nonfat vanilla Greek yogurt

PB&J Overnight Oats
- ½ cup (83 g) sliced strawberries
- 1 heaping tablespoon (17 g) peanut butter (plus more for drizzling on top, if desired)
- 1 tablespoon (14 g) chia seeds
- 2 scoops unflavored collagen powder (1 serving)

Chunky Monkey Overnight Oats
- ½ banana, mashed
- 1 tablespoon (17 g) crunchy or smooth peanut butter
- 1 tablespoon (7.5 g) chopped walnuts
- 1 to 2 tablespoon (10 to 20 g) chocolate chips or 1 scoop chocolate protein powder

Apple Cinnamon Overnight Oats
- 1 medium Granny Smith Apple, chopped and divided
- 2 tablespoons (20 g) hemp seeds
- 1 teaspoon cinnamon

You Will Need
- Mason jar or other container with lid or bowl with plastic wrap or beeswax wrap
- Liquid measuring cup
- ½-cup measuring cup
- Measuring spoons

Instructions

1. Add base ingredients and variation ingredients to a mason jar and seal it with a lid. Shake the jar to combine the ingredients.

2. Place the jar in the fridge to chill for at least 3 hours, but ideally overnight.

Notes
- If using a bowl, use a spoon to mix and cover with beeswax or plastic wrap.

Mixed Berry Chia Pudding

Chia seeds may be small, but they are a nutrition powerhouse. They are a great source of alpha-linolenic acid (ALA), a plant-based omega-3, and provide about 10 grams of fiber per serving (2½ tablespoons). Their mild flavor makes them a great ingredient to sprinkle into smoothies, overnight oats, pancakes, cereal, and even yogurt. If you want a prep-in-advance breakfast or snack, this simple mixed berry chia pudding is a great option.

Yield: 2 servings

Ingredients

- 1 cup (236 ml) unsweetened vanilla oat milk or milk of choice
- 1 teaspoon honey
- ½ cup (70 g) frozen mixed berries
- 1 serving or 2 scoops unflavored collagen powder (may vary by brand)
- 1 teaspoon lemon juice
- ¼ cup (40 g) chia seeds

Optional toppings: hemp seeds, Greek or coconut yogurt, fresh berries, sliced almonds, nut or seed butter, chopped walnuts

You Will Need

- Blender or food processor
- Liquid measuring cup
- ½-cup measuring cup
- ¼-cup measuring cup
- Measuring spoons
- Two 16-ounce mason jars with lids or other airtight containers

Instructions

1. Add milk, honey, frozen mixed berries, collagen powder, and lemon juice to a blender or food processor. Blend on high for 1 to 2 minutes or until smooth.

2. Add the chia seeds. Switch the blender to low and blend until the chia seeds are just mixed in, approximately 15 to 20 seconds.

3. Divide the pudding between two 16-ounce mason jars or other sealable containers. Tightly seal the lid and refrigerate for at least 4 hours or overnight.

4. Garnish with your favorite toppings and enjoy straight from container.

NOTE: You can store these in the fridge for 5 to 6 days. You could double or triple this recipe if needed. If you want to add more protein, top with Greek yogurt, hemp seeds, or nuts.

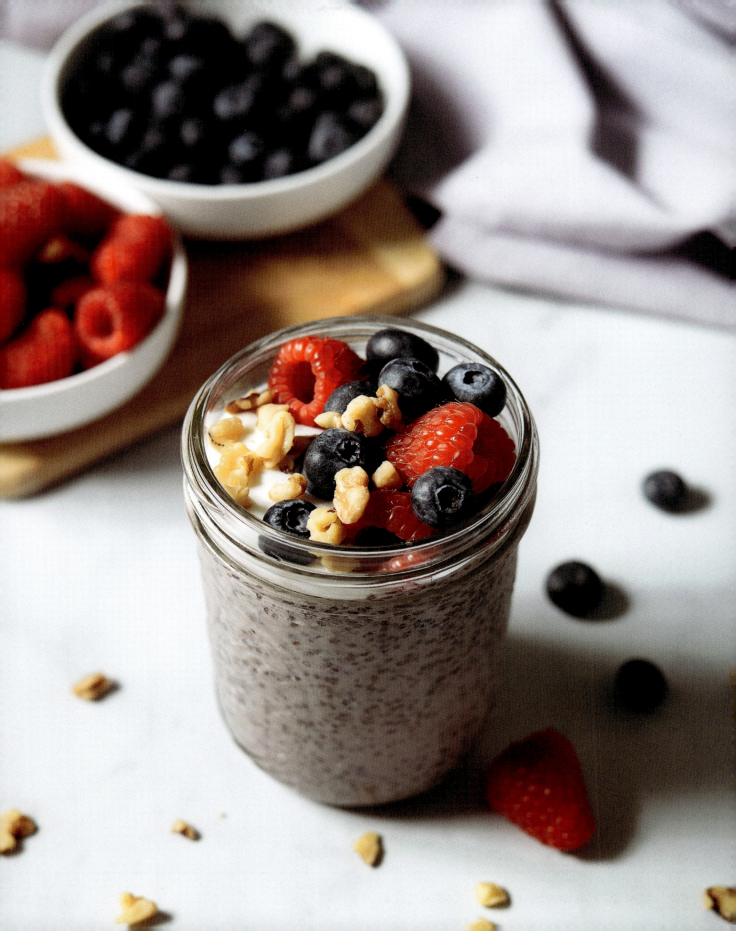

Avocado Toast with Fried Egg

Avocados are a great source of monounsaturated fats, potassium, and fiber. When I make avocado toast, I like to add extra spices to my avocado for more flavor. I also mix in chia seeds for a little extra healthy fat and fiber to help me feel fuller for longer. Feel free to use store-bought mashed avocado cups if you don't want to waste time mashing and seasoning your avocado.

Yield: 1 serving

Ingredients

- 1 large egg
- 2 slices of high-fiber bread
- 1 small avocado or half of a medium size avocado
- 2 teaspoons chia seeds
- ½ teaspoon smoked paprika
- ½ teaspoon turmeric
- Salt and pepper to taste
- ½ teaspoon Everything Bagel Seasoning
- Sriracha (optional)

You Will Need

- Cooking spray
- Small nonstick pan
- Toaster or oven
- Knife
- Small bowl
- Measuring spoons
- Fork
- Spatula

Instructions

1. Heat a small, nonstick pan on medium-high heat. Spray the pan with cooking spray.

2. Once the pan is heated, crack the egg in the pan. Fry egg until the white is set and the yolk is slightly white, about 3 minutes. Gently flip the egg and leave in pan for about 30 seconds for an over-easy fried egg before transferring to a plate.

3. While the egg is frying, toast bread to desired doneness. Slice the avocado in half and remove the pit. Squeeze the meat of the avocado into the bowl and discard the skin. Add the chia seeds, paprika, turmeric, salt, and pepper to the bowl. Use a fork to mash up the avocado.

4. Place toast on the plate with the egg. Use a fork or spatula to spread the mashed avocado on the toast. Top with Everything Bagel Seasoning and Sriracha. Enjoy!

Breakfast Tacos

This is one of my favorite ways to use up leftovers from my fajita bowl meal (see page 155). Just add scrambled eggs and you've got delicious breakfast tacos! I prefer to use high-fiber tortillas in this recipe because it's an easy way to work in extra fiber, and I don't notice a difference. If you don't have fajita leftovers, just sauté a little frozen pepper and onion blend and season it with fajita seasoning before cooking the eggs.

Yield: 1 serving

Ingredients
- 2 large eggs
- 2 tablespoons (30 ml) milk
- ¼ cup (25 g) shredded Mexican cheese
- Salt and pepper, to taste
- 1 tablespoon (14 g) butter
- ½ cup (115 g) leftover fajita steak and veggies
- 2 street taco-sized tortillas
- 2 tablespoons (28 g) guacamole, divided
- 2 tablespoons (28 g) salsa, divided
- 2 tablespoons (28 g) sour cream, optional

You Will Need
- Small mixing bowl
- ¼-cup and ½-cup measuring cups
- Measuring spoons
- Fork or whisk
- Medium nonstick pan
- Microwave-safe plate
- Damp paper towel
- Rubber spatula

Instructions

1. Crack the eggs into a bowl. Add milk and shredded cheese, salt, and pepper. Use a fork or whisk to scramble the eggs, mixing until everything is combined.

2. Place a medium, nonstick pan on medium heat. Add butter to pan. Once it is melted, add leftover fajita mix. Cook for 3 to 5 minutes to heat leftovers.

3. While the fajita mixture heats up, place the tortilla on a microwave safe plate and cover with a damp paper towel. Microwave for 15 to 20 seconds.

4. Push fajita mix to one half of the pan to keep warm. Turn heat to medium-low. In the other half of the pan, pour the egg mixture and wait 30 seconds until the edges begin to set. Use a rubber spatula to push eggs from one end of pan to the other, keeping them separate from the fajita mix. After 2 to 3 minutes, large, soft curds will form. The eggs are done when they are set, but still a little runny.

5. Remove the tortillas from the microwave. Set aside the paper towel and separate the tortillas, if needed. Add a shmear of guacamole to each tortilla and top with half the egg and fajita mix. Top with salsa and sour cream. Enjoy!

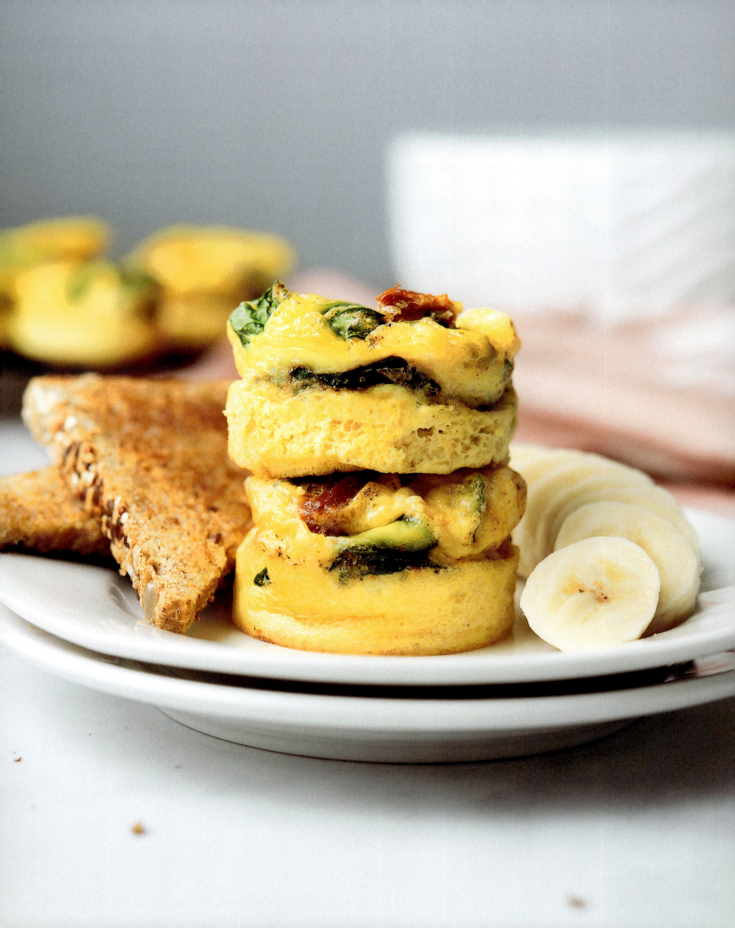

Egg Bites, Three Ways

Egg bites are a great make-in-advance breakfast, and this is my favorite way to make them. If you like omelets, you can use your favorite toppings in your own egg bites or follow one of my three recipe variations below. Note that you may need to adjust the toppings if making more than one kind in a batch.

Yield: 12 egg bites or 6 servings (see note)

Ingredients

Egg Bite Base
- 12 large eggs
- ¼ cup (60 ml) milk
- Salt and pepper to taste

Spinach and Feta Egg Bites
- 1 cup (100 g) spinach, roughly chopped
- ½ cup (57 g) feta cheese
- ¼ cup (14 g) sun-dried tomatoes
- ½ teaspoon garlic powder

Ham and Cheese Egg Bites
- ¾ cup (113 g) chopped baked or deli ham
- ⅔ cup (67 g) shredded Gruyere cheese
- ¼ cup (36 g) onion, diced

Veggie-Packed Egg Bites
- ½ cup (71 g) red onion, diced
- ½ cup (71 g) red bell pepper, diced
- ¼ cup (22 g) broccoli, finely chopped
- 1 cup (100 g) shredded mozzarella cheese

You Will Need
- 1 12-count muffin pan
- Cooking spray or silicone muffin cups
- Large mixing bowl
- Liquid measuring cup
- ¼-, ⅓-, and ½-cup measuring cups
- Measuring spoons
- Whisk or fork
- Oven mitt
- Food thermometer

Instructions

1. Preheat oven to 350°F (177°C). Coat a 12-count muffin tin with nonstick cooking spray or line with silicone muffin cups.

2. In a large mixing bowl, beat eggs, milk, salt, and pepper until combined. Add the other ingredients from your variation of choice and whisk to combine.

3. Divide egg mixture between 12 muffin cups, making sure not to fill the cups more than three-quarters of the way full. Bake for 15 to 17 minutes, or until the center of the egg cups are set and no longer shiny on top. The internal temperature should be 165°F (74°C). Remove from the oven and let them cool for a few minutes before removing them from the cups.

4. Enjoy warm! Optional: To store, wrap each muffin in plastic wrap (optional) and place in a resealable bag. Store in refrigerator for up to 6 days and freezer for 3 months. To reheat, unwrap from plastic wrap and then wrap in a damp paper towel. Microwave on a plate for 20-second increments until heated through.

Notes: Suggested serving size is 2 egg bites. You may want to pair them with a carb like an English muffin, toast, biscuit, or banana.

High-Protein Pancakes with Berries

Protein pancakes are great for ADHDers who may struggle to get enough protein at the beginning of the day but want a sweeter breakfast. I like to use a protein pancake mix so I don't have to measure a bunch of ingredients or use a blender, which also makes for fewer dishes. You can make these with milk for even more protein or water if you want to make this dairy-free.

Yield: Makes 6 4-inch (10 cm) pancakes

Ingredients

- 1 cup (120 g) protein pancake mix
- ¾ cup (177 ml) 2% milk or water
- 1 teaspoon cinnamon (optional)
- Cooking spray
- ¼ cup (60 g) almond butter
- 1 cup (150 g) frozen mixed berries
- ¼ cup (28 g) granola (optional crunch factor)

You Will Need

- Medium mixing bowl
- ¼- and 1-cup measuring cups
- Liquid measuring cup
- Measuring spoons
- Mixing spoon
- Medium nonstick pan
- Spatula
- 2 small microwave-safe bowls
- Fork

Instructions

1. In a medium mixing bowl, add protein pancake mix, milk or water, and cinnamon. Stir until just combined; do not overmix.

2. Spray the pan with cooking spray and heat over medium-high heat. Use the measuring cup to scoop about ¼ cup of batter and pour it into the heated pan. Cook pancake until you see bubbles start to form, about 1 to 2 minutes. Flip the pancake and continue cooking until golden brown, about 1 to 2 minutes. Repeat with remaining batter.

3. While the pancakes cook, place the almond butter in a microwave safe bowl. Microwave for about 10 seconds or until the almond butter is warm and runny. Place the frozen mixed berries in a separate microwave safe bowl. Microwave berries for seconds. Remove berries and use a fork to mash them in the bowl. Microwave for another 10 to seconds, if desired. Berries should be thawed and gooey.

4. Divide pancakes between two plates. Top each with half of melted almond butter and mixed berries.

Berry Blast Smoothie

I make this smoothie, or some version of it, often. The mixed berries are an excellent source of vitamin C, antioxidants, and fiber. And blending the fruit doesn't remove the fiber as it does when you juice it.

Yield: 1 smoothie

Ingredients

- 1 cup (237 ml) unsweetened vanilla almond milk
- 1 cup (163 g) frozen mixed berries
- ½ medium frozen banana
- 1 scoop or serving vanilla protein powder of your choice
- 1 tablespoon (7 g) ground flaxseed
- 1 teaspoon cinnamon (optional)

You Will Need

- Blender
- Liquid measuring cup
- ½-cup and 1-cup measuring cups
- Measuring spoons

Instructions

1. Add all ingredients to the blender, starting with the liquid (this makes it easier to blend). Place lid on the blender and blend on high until smooth. Pour into a glass and enjoy!

General Smoothie Tips:

- Add-ins that incorporate protein and fat are a must if you want your smoothie to keep you full. A few ideas are protein powder, chia seeds, ground flaxseed, nut butter, avocado, tofu, Greek yogurt, and cottage cheese.
- Consider a blender that has cup attachments for easier clean up. Or to clean a blender pitcher, add warm soapy water, place lid back on, and run for 1 to 2 minutes.
- Prep frozen and dry ingredients in a reusable sealable bag. This allows you to just dump the contents of the bag into the blender and add the liquid when it's time to make the smoothie.
- Use less liquid for a thicker smoothie.

Strawberry Peanut Butter Smoothie

This is a protein powder-free smoothie! The protein in it comes from the vanilla Greek yogurt, with peanut butter powder for an extra boost.

Yield: 1 smoothie

Ingredients
- 1 cup (237 ml) 2% milk or liquid of your choice
- 1 cup (163 g) frozen strawberries
- ½ cup (122 g) vanilla Greek yogurt
- 2 tablespoons (34 g) peanut butter powder or regular peanut butter
- 2 teaspoons ground flaxseed

You Will Need
- Blender
- Liquid measuring cup
- ½-cup and 1-cup measuring cups
- Measuring spoons

Instructions
1. Add all ingredients to a blender starting with the liquid. Place lid on the blender and blend on high until smooth. Pour into a glass and enjoy!

Note: You can find peanut butter powder online or in the same aisle as peanut butter at the grocery store.

Tropical Paradise Smoothie

I use collagen powder in this smoothie, but you can use a flavorless protein powder of your choice.

Yield: 1 smoothie

Ingredients
- 1¼ cup (313 g) unsweetened vanilla almond milk or liquid of choice
- 1 cup (163 g) frozen tropical fruit blend
- 1 serving collagen powder
- 2 teaspoons chia seeds

You Will Need
- Blender
- Liquid measuring cup
- ½-cup and 1-cup measuring cups
- Measuring spoons

Instructions
1. Add all ingredients to a blender, starting with the liquid. Place lid on the blender and blend on high until smooth. Pour into a glass and enjoy!

Cold Brew Smoothie

This smoothie is my reverse-engineered version of one of my favorite Clean Juice smoothies, though I use date syrup because dates don't blend well and would clog up my straw. It does require some slight prepping in advance; the cold brew concentrate has to be frozen in ice cube trays the night before. This, plus the frozen banana, help make the smoothie thick and creamy. I personally enjoy oat milk or 2-percent milk in this smoothie, but feel free to use your milk of choice.

Yield: 1 smoothie

Ingredients

- 1 cup (237 ml) milk of choice
- 6 to 8 frozen cold brew concentrate cubes (see notes)
- 1 banana, roughly chopped and frozen
- 2 tablespoons (34 g) almond butter
- 1 teaspoon date syrup or honey

You Will Need

- Blender
- Liquid measuring cup
- ½-cup and 1-cup measuring cups
- Measuring spoons
- Ice cube tray

Instructions

1. Add all ingredients to a blender, starting with the liquid. Place lid on the blender and blend on high until smooth. Pour into a glass and enjoy!

Notes: To make the cold brew concentrate cubes, fill an ice cube tray with the cold brew concentrate. I use a 15-cube silicone ice cube tray. Place in the freezer for at least 6 hours or until frozen.

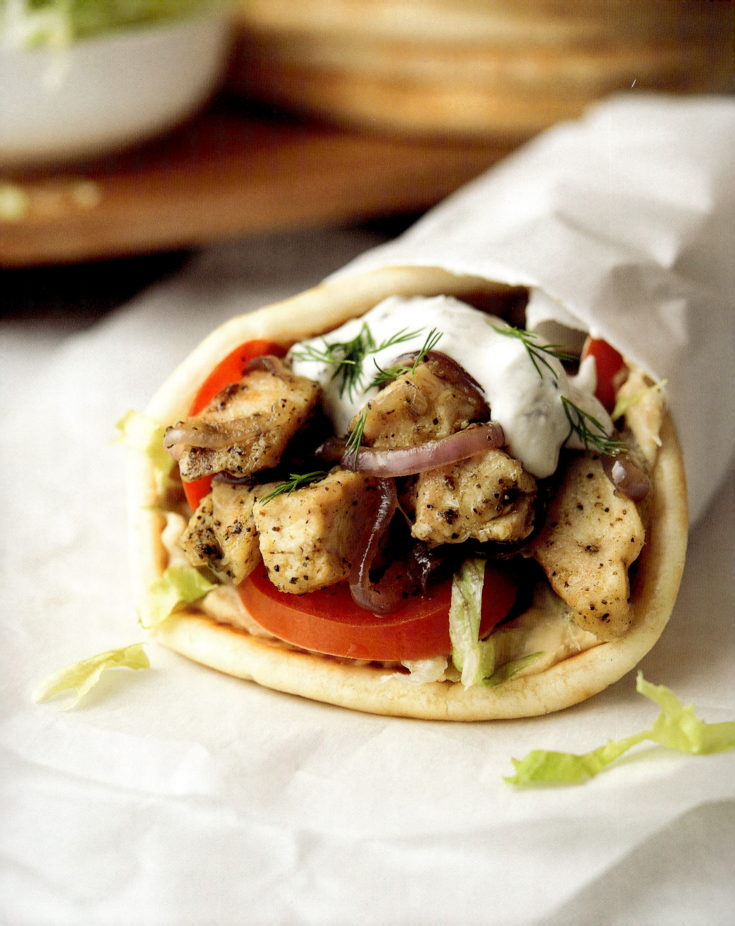

Chicken Gyro Wrap

I love making this on my lunch break because it comes together so fast. You could also prep the veggies and cook the chicken in advance and assemble later. Feel free to use frozen, precooked grilled chicken, store-bought hummus, and tzatziki to save some time and energy.

Yield: 2 servings

Ingredients

- ½ pound (227 g) chicken tenderloins, cut into ½-inch (1 cm) pieces
- 3 tablespoons (45 ml) olive oil, divided
- 1 to 2 ounces (28 to 57 g) All-Purpose Greek seasoning
- ½ red onion, sliced
- 2 Mediterranean pitas
- 4 ounces (113.5 g) hummus or tzatziki
- 1 plum tomato, thinly sliced
- ½ cup (35 g) pre-shredded lettuce

You Will Need

- Paper towel
- Measuring spoons
- Large mixing bowl
- Medium nonstick pan
- Tongs or spatula
- Food thermometer
- Cutting board
- Knife
- ½-cup measuring cup

Instructions

1. Pat the chicken dry with a paper towel. Add chicken, 1 tablespoon (15 ml) olive oil, Greek seasoning, salt and pepper to a mixing bowl and toss until chicken is well coated.

2. Heat a medium nonstick pan over medium-high heat. Add 1 tablespoon (15 ml) of olive oil and heat until oil is shimmering. Add the chicken and onions and cook, stirring occasionally, until the chicken is browned and onions are tender, about 7 to 9 minutes. Chicken should have an internal temp of 165°F (74°C).

3. Preheat broiler on high and make sure the rack is in the top position. Brush each side of the pitas with 1 tablespoon (15 ml) of olive oil. Place pitas on rack. Cook for 1 to 2 minutes per side. DO NOT STEP AWAY FROM OVEN while the pitas are under the broiler. You may need to stare at it like a little kid. Pitas should be warm, slightly browned, and pliable—not burnt.

4. Spread hummus or tzatziki on one side of your pitas. Top with tomatoes and chicken and onion mixture. Wrap like a burrito or fold in half like a taco and enjoy!

Walking "Tacos"

This is a fun way to incorporate your favorite chips into a meal. I like to make these when I have leftover taco meat. I use lean ground turkey to cut down on the saturated fat content, but you are welcome to use ground beef or tofu. The fun part about these is that you can customize them. We usually serve this taco bar-style, setting out all the toppings so each of us can make our own. Instead of using bowls, we usually serve the toppings in glass storage containers so we can put the lids on and stash them in the fridge for later.

Yield: 4 servings

Ingredients

- 1 pound (453 g) 93% lean ground turkey
- 1 taco seasoning packet
- ⅔ cup (157 ml) water
- 4 single-serving bags of chips such as Fritos, Doritos, tortilla chips
- 1 [8-ounce (226 g)] bag of shredded lettuce
- ½ cup (50 g) shredded Mexican-blend cheese or cheese of our choice
- ½ cup (124 g) pico de gallo
- Sour cream
- 1 jalapeño pepper, thinly sliced

You Will Need

- Medium nonstick pan
- Liquid measuring cup
- Spatula or wooden spoon
- Cutting board
- Knife
- ½-cup measuring cup

Instructions

1. Heat a medium pan over medium-high heat until hot. Add ground turkey and cook, breaking it up with a spatula or wooden spoon until it is mostly brown and cooked through, approximately 10 minutes.

2. Add packet of taco seasoning and water to the pan and stir to combine. Reduce the heat to low and simmer for 3 to 5 minutes or until the sauce has thickened.

3. Thinly slice the jalapeño pepper.

4. Open the bags of chips and divide the taco meat evenly between the four bags. Top with lettuce, cheese, pico de gallo, sour cream, and jalapeños slices. Enjoy straight out of the bag!

Build Your Own ADHD Charcuterie Plate or Board

Before the TikTok "girl dinner" trend, I referred to a plate of snacks or finger foods as "ADHD charcuterie." Sometimes you just want a little bit of a lot of different foods that you can enjoy with your hands. If you want to make your ADHD charcuterie plate or board not only satisfying to your tastebuds, but also a meal that fills you up, follow the formula below. Don't hesitate to add more food if you need to, depending on your hunger levels.

In the table on page 144, I've categorized charcuterie ingredients based on which macronutrient each one contains the most of. When building your plate, pick higher fiber carbs to help you stay full for longer. If you pick simple carbs, you might want to add more high fiber fruits or veggies such as berries or broccoli. Think of the satisfaction factor as anything you can add to your plate, that makes it more enjoyable or gets you excited about eating. These ingredients are fun little add-ons to your basic plate.

One of the cool things about these plates is that you can mix and match to meet your sensory needs. This is also a great way to incorporate leftovers that you don't quite have enough of to make a full meal—add them to a plate with whatever else is missing (carbs, protein, fat) and you've got dinner.

I've included some sample plates to get you started. Enjoy!

Sample ADHD Charcuterie Plate 1

Protein: canned tuna

Carb: flaxseed crackers

Fat: avocado slices and walnuts

Volume: carrot sticks and apple

Satisfaction factor: pickles and dark chocolate square

Sample ADHD Charcuterie Plate 2 (Vegan)

Protein: hummus

Carb: whole wheat pita bread and dried figs

Fat: olives

Volume: grapes, cucumber sticks, and radishes

Satisfaction factor: Vegan cookie

Sample ADHD Charcuterie Plate 3

Protein: smoked salmon and hard-boiled egg

Carb: crostini

Fat: cream cheese

Veggies: cucumber slices and cherry tomatoes

Satisfaction factor: capers

Build Your Own ADHD Charcuterie Formula

Yield: 1 serving

1 to 2 proteins	1 to 2 carbohydrates	1 to 2 fats	1 to 2 volume foods (fruits and/or veggies)	1 to 2 foods for the "satisfaction factor"
Protein	**Carbohydrate**	**Fat**	**Volume**	**Satisfaction Factor**
Deli meat	Crackers	Nuts (almonds, walnuts, cashews, peanuts, etc.)	Apple slices	Artisanal jams
Hard-boiled eggs	Tortilla chips		Banana	Honey
Smoked salmon	Pretzels		Grapes	Dijon mustard
Canned tuna or sardines	Whole wheat pita bread	Pumpkin seeds	Berries	Pickles
Edamame	Pasta	Olives	Carrots	Pickled veggies
Hummus	Bread	Nut butter	Baby cucumber	Nutella
Cottage cheese	Beans	Avocado slices	Mini peppers or bell pepper slices	Whole grain mustard
Cheese	Dried snap peas	Guacamole	Radishes	Capers
Rotisserie chicken	Plantain chips	Garlic dip	Clementine	Anything sweet
Beef or turkey jerky	Pita chips	Ranch dressing	Cherry tomatoes	
Dried chickpeas	Popcorn	Tapenade	Sugar snap peas	
Lupini beans	Granola	Tahini sauce	Dates	
Kielbasa sausage	Dried fruits (figs, apricots, raisins)	Cream cheese	Kiwi	
Chicken nuggets	Crostini		Pineapple	
Greek yogurt			Peaches	
Tempeh			Broccoli	
Lentils			Green peas	
Charcuterie (prosciutto, salami, chorizo, soppressata, ham, cured sausages)			Zucchini	

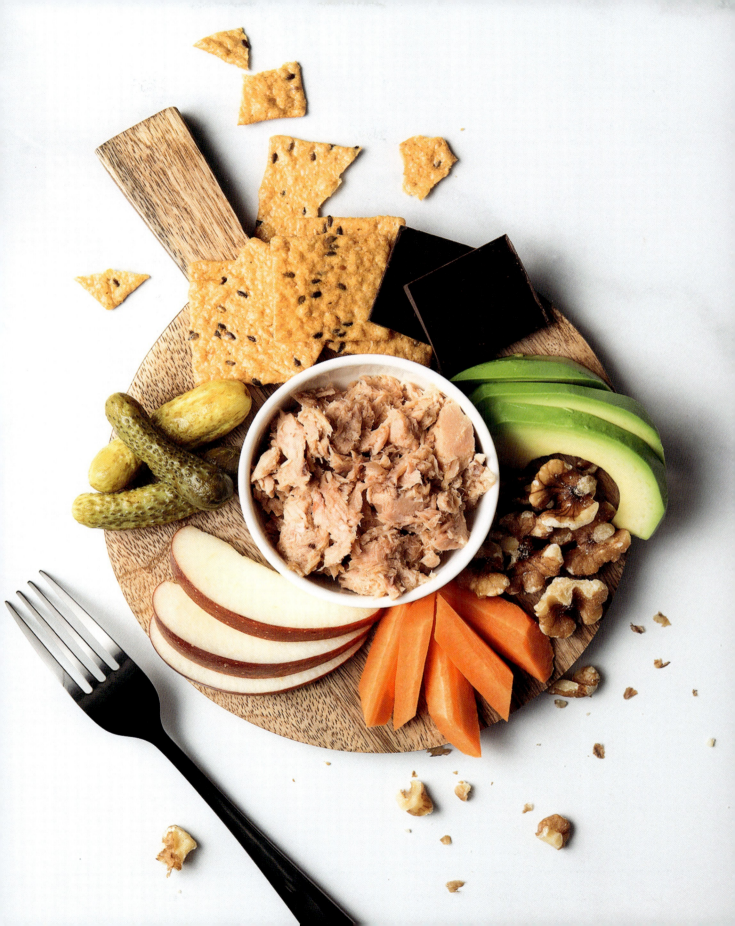

Buffalo Chicken Wrap

One of my hyperfixation flavors is buffalo. This wrap is a go-to lunch when all I want to do is cover everything I eat with buffalo sauce. I add crunchy veggies for the crunch factor. You can use store-bought ranch dressing, but I like to use Greek yogurt and Ranch seasoning for a little extra protein. This wrap can easily be turned into a salad if that's what you'd prefer! You can do this by using shredded lettuce as the base and top with the crunchy veggies, buffalo chicken mixture, and some extra ranch dressing.

Yield: 1 wrap

Ingredients
- 1 cup (125 g) shredded rotisserie chicken
- ¼ cup (57 g) buffalo sauce
- ¼ cup (65 g) Greek yogurt
- 1 heaping teaspoon ranch seasoning
- Tortillas
- ½ cup (72 g) shredded lettuce
- ½ cup (71 g) shredded carrots
- 1 to 2 green onions, thinly sliced

You Will Need
- Medium mixing bowl
- ½-cup measuring cup
- Knife
- Measuring spoons
- Cutting board

Instructions

1. In a medium bowl, combine shredded chicken, buffalo sauce, Greek yogurt, and ranch seasoning. Mix until combined.

2. Lay tortilla on a plate. Place half of mixture in the center of the tortilla. Top with lettuce, carrots, and green onion. Fold opposite sides of the tortilla toward the middle. Then, fold the side closest to you toward the middle and roll up to turn it into a wrap.

Italian Pasta Salad

My partner and I love making a big batch of a cold salad to keep in the fridge for an easy snack or meal, especially during the hot Southern summers. If you like an Italian sub, you'll enjoy this pasta salad. I use protein pasta to boost the protein. If you need a gluten-free option, try Banza or Barilla's chickpea or red lentil rotini pasta. If you don't like any of these veggies, feel free to leave them out. I always give my partner the black olives!

Yield: 6 large servings

Ingredients

- 1 [14.5-ounce (411 g)] box of rotini protein pasta
- ½ cup (70 g) Salami, chopped
- ½ cup (70 g) pepperoni, chopped
- ¼ cup (60 g) sliced banana peppers
- 1 cup (142 g) diced green bell pepper
- 1 [12-ounce (340 g)] jar roasted red peppers
- 1 pint cherry tomatoes, halved
- 8 ounces (227 g) Mozzarella pearls (1 package)
- ½ cup (58 g) red onion, diced
- 1 2.25-ounce (64 g) can sliced black olives.
- 1 cup (236 ml) Italian salad dressing, divided

You Will Need

- Medium pot
- Colander
- Large mixing bowl
- Large spoon
- ¼-cup and ½-cup measuring cups
- Knife
- Cutting board
- Measuring spoon
- Plastic wrap

Instructions

1. Bring 6 cups (1.4 L) of water to boil in a medium pot over high heat. Follow directions on the box to cook protein pasta.

2. As the pasta cooks, cut up the meats and vegetables.

3. Drain the pasta in a colander and dump it into a large mixing bowl. Let cool for at least 15 minutes. Do not rinse the pasta.

4. When the pasta is cool, add ½ cup (118 ml) of Italian dressing and the remaining ingredients to the mixing bowl with the pasta. Toss with a large spoon to evenly coat the pasta, vegetables, and meats with the dressing. Cover with plastic wrap and refrigerate for at least 3 hours. Add the remaining dressing just before serving.

5. Store any remaining pasta salad in an airtight container for up to 3 days.

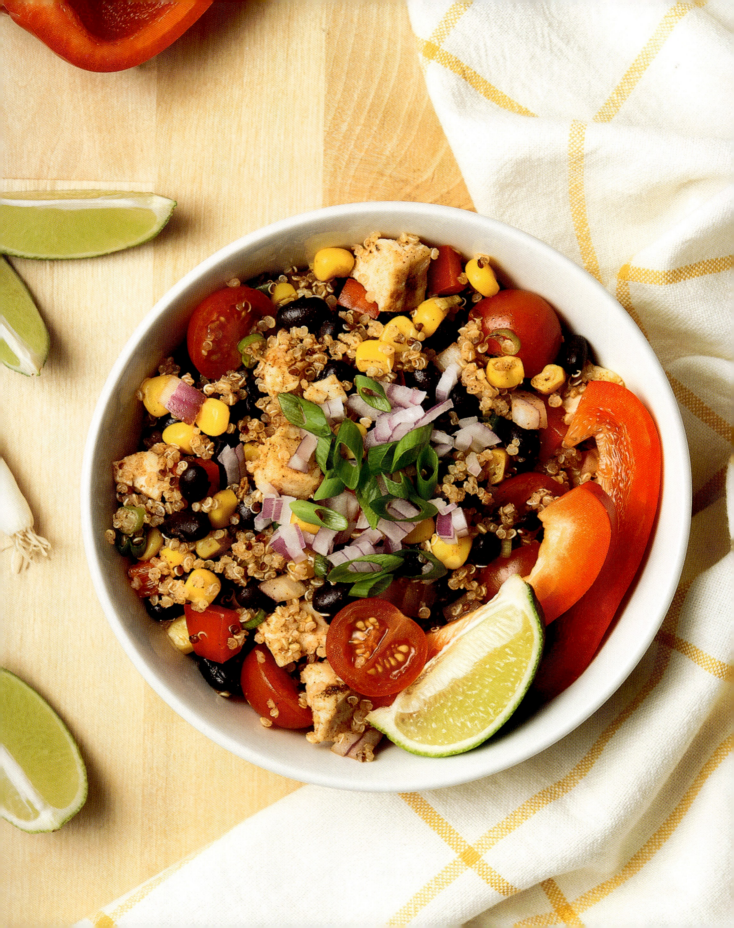

Southwestern Quinoa Salad

This was one of my go-to meals in undergrad and grad school because you can enjoy it hot or cold. Quinoa is a versatile, gluten-free grain, that provides 8 grams of protein and 5 grams of fiber in a one-cup serving. For plant-based folks, it is considered a "complete protein" because it provides all nine essential amino acids, which means you don't need to combine it with other foods to get all the protein you need. You can save a few steps in this recipe by using frozen pre-cooked chicken cubes, pre-chopped peppers and onion, and a couple 90-second microwavable pre-cooked quinoa pouches. You can customize this recipe with whatever toppings you'd like. If you are plant-based, you could swap the pre-cooked chicken for tofu crumbles or nothing—without the chicken this meal will provide 16 grams of protein per serving.

Yield: 2 servings

Ingredients
- 1 cup (185 g) quinoa
- ½ cup (75 g) chopped red bell pepper
- ½ cup (75 g) chopped red onion
- 1 cup (150 g) cherry tomatoes, sliced
- 2 scallions, thinly sliced
- 2 tablespoons (30 ml) olive oil, divided
- 8 ounces (224 g) frozen precooked chicken tenderloins (4 frozen tenders)
- 1 8.75-ounce can (241 g) sweet whole kernel corn, canned, drained
- 1 [15.25-ounce (432 g)] can black beans, drained and rinsed
- 1 tablespoon (15 ml) lime juice
- ½ low-sodium taco seasoning packet
- ½ to 1 teaspoon salt (depending on taste)

Optional: guacamole, salsa, sour cream, sliced jalapeño peppers

You Will Need
- Mesh strainer
- Medium pot
- 1-cup measuring cup
- Liquid measuring cup
- Fork
- Large mixing bowl
- Measuring spoons
- Medium pan
- Spatula
- Cutting board
- Utility knife
- Can opener

Instructions

1. Check the directions on the quinoa packaging to see if it needs to be rinsed before cooking. If so, rinse in a mesh strainer. In a medium pot, combine the quinoa and 2 cups (474 ml) water. Bring to a boil, cover, reduce the heat to low, and simmer for 15 minutes or until light, fluffy, and tender. Remove from the heat and let it sit, covered, for an additional 10 minutes. Fluff with fork.

2. Chop the bell pepper, onion, tomatoes, and scallions, add them to the large mixing bowl, and set aside.

3. Add 1 tablespoon (15 ml) olive oil to a medium pan and set over medium-high heat.

4. When the oil is shimmering, add the chicken to the pan. Cook until the chicken is heated to 165°F (74°C), turning to cook all sides. Remove the chicken from the pan and let cool on cutting board for 10 minutes. Roughly chop into ½-inch (1-cm) pieces.

5. Add cooked quinoa, chicken, beans, corn, remaining olive oil, lime juice, half of the taco seasoning packet, and salt to the large mixing bowl with the chopped veggies. Stir.

6. Serve in a bowl with your favorite toppings, such as guacamole, salsa, sour cream, and sliced jalapeños and enjoy! Store leftovers in an airtight container and eat within 5 days.

Salmon Sheet Pan with Roasted Veggies and Potatoes

Salmon contains the type of omega-3s that are important for ADHD brains, so this is an excellent recipe to have in your weekly rotation. To save time and energy, this recipe uses a pre-seasoned salmon filet, which you can find at many grocery stores (I like the Mediterranean herb salmon from ALDI). I also try to buy my Brussels sprouts already halved so I don't have to chop anything. If you want to eat this meal every week to get your omega-3s, add some variety by swapping out the veggies for broccoli, asparagus, zucchini, and tomatoes, or a combination of them!

Yield: 4 servings

Ingredients

- 1½ pounds (680 g) red baby potatoes, rinsed and dried
- 2 tablespoons (30 ml) olive oil, divided
- 2 tablespoons (30 ml) balsamic vinegar, divided
- 1 tablespoon (6 g) Italian seasoning, divided
- 1 tablespoon (8 g) minced garlic, divided
- 1 [12-ounce (340 g)] bag halved Brussels sprouts
- Salt and pepper to taste
- 1 [1-pound (453 g)] pre-seasoned salmon filet

You Will Need

- Cooking spray
- Silicone baking mat or parchment paper
- Sheet pan
- Large bowl
- Spoon
- Spatula
- Knife
- Measuring spoons

Instructions

1. Preheat oven to 400°F (204°C). Line a sheet pan with a silicone baking mat or parchment paper and set aside.

2. Add red potatoes to a large bowl and drizzle with 1 tablespoon (15 ml) olive oil and 1 tablespoon (15 ml) balsamic vinegar. Use a spoon to toss the potatoes until they're well coated. Add ½ tablespoon Italian seasoning, ½ tablespoon minced garlic, and salt and pepper to taste. Mix again until seasoning is evenly distributed.

3. Pour the potatoes onto the sheet pan and place the pan in the oven. Set a timer for 15 minutes and let them cook.

4. While the potatoes cook, add the Brussels sprouts to the same mixing bowl and toss with the remaining olive oil, balsamic vinegar, Italian seasoning, and garlic. Add salt and pepper to taste.

5. When the timer goes off, remove the sheet pan from the oven and push the potatoes to one side of pan. Add salmon to the middle of the pan and the Brussels sprouts to the other side.

6. Place the sheet pan back in oven for to 20 to 25 minutes or until the salmon is cooked to 145°F (63°C) and the Brussels sprouts and potatoes are slightly crispy. If needed, set oven to the broiler setting, remove the salmon, and cook the vegetables for 2 to 3 additional minutes until they are extra crispy.

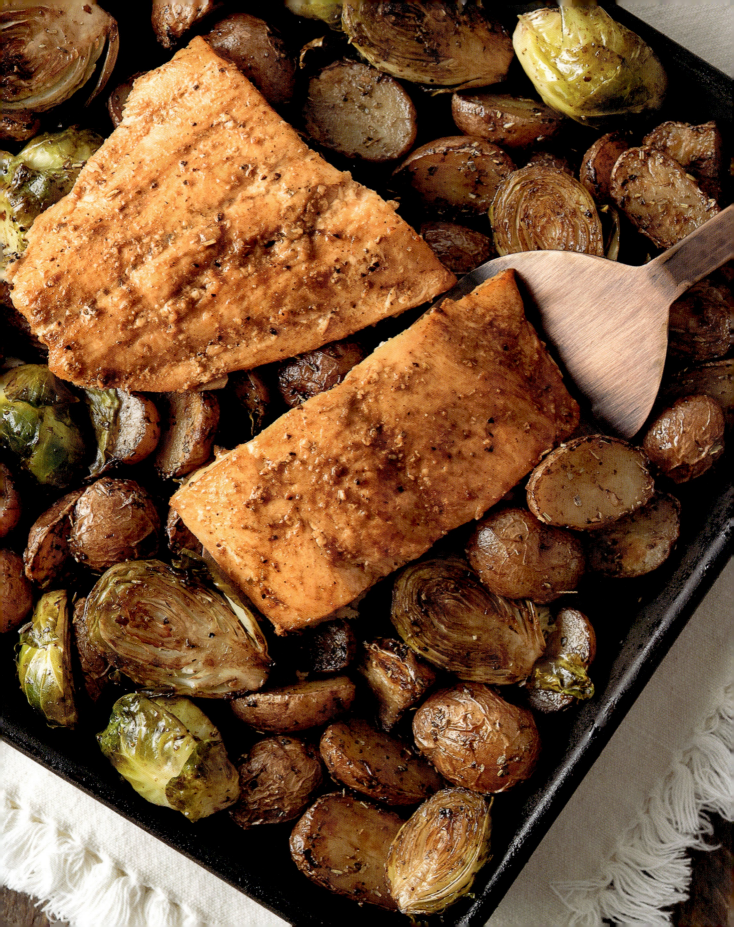

Mediterranean Meatballs and Chickpea Orzo

This meal is super flavorful and quick. I used precooked roasted garlic chicken meatballs and Banza chickpea orzo, because it has more fiber and protein than regular orzo.

Yield: 2 servings

Ingredients

- 3 tablespoons (45 ml) olive oil, divided
- 1 [10-ounce (283 g)] package of fully cooked roasted garlic chicken meatballs
- Salt
- ½ cup (100 g) chickpea orzo
- ¼ cup (50 g) sliced kalamata olives
- 1 baby cucumber, sliced and halved
- 10 cherry tomatoes, halved
- 2 teaspoons Italian seasoning
- ¼ cup (61 g) feta cheese crumbles

You Will Need

- Medium saucepan
- Measuring spoons
- Measuring cup
- Fine mesh strainer
- Wooden spoon

Instructions

1. In a medium saucepan, add 2 tablespoons (30 ml) olive oil and place over medium heat. Add the meatballs and cook for about 3 minutes or until heated through. Transfer to a plate and cover.

2. In the same saucepan, bring 6 cups (1.4 L) of salted water to a rolling boil. Reduce heat to a simmer and add orzo. Cook until desired firmness or about 5 minutes. Stir occasionally.

3. As the orzo cooks, chop the cucumber and cherry tomatoes. Set aside.

4. Once the orzo is cooked, use a fine mesh strainer to drain it and rinse well. Add the orzo, olives, cucumber, tomatoes, Italian seasoning, and remaining olive oil to the saucepan. Toss to combine.

5. Serve meatballs and orzo together in a bowl.

Spicy Pickle Flatbread

If you're like me and will gladly take someone else's pickle, you need to try this flatbread. It's the perfect mix of salty and spicy. You can totally use pre-shredded cheese, but I prefer to shred it myself because pre-shredded cheese has potato starch in it. This prevents the cheese from clumping in the package, but can also prevent the cheese from turning into melty goodness when it's cooked. I like to eat pizza or flatbread with either a side salad or carrots and ranch to add some fiber so I will feel fuller for longer.

Yield: 2 servings

Ingredients

Ranch Sauce
- ½ cup (130 g) plain nonfat Greek yogurt
- ¼ cup (56 g) mayonnaise
- 1 1-ounce (28 g) packet of ranch seasoning

Flatbread
- 1 (220 g) frozen store-bought Flatbread
- 1 cup (153 g) jarred dill pickle slices, patted dry, divided (you can use more if you'd like)
- 1 cup (115 g) low-moisture mozzarella, shredded
- ½ cup (58 g) provolone cheese, shredded
- ⅔ cup (90 g) rotisserie chicken, shredded
- 1 teaspoon dried dill, divided
- 2 tablespoons (30 ml) store-bought hot honey

You Will Need
- Small bowl
- Mixing spoon
- Rubber spatula
- Paper towels
- ¼-cup, ⅓-cup, and ½-cup measuring cups
- Measuring spoons
- Scissors or pizza cutter

Instructions

1. Preheat oven to 425°F (218°C) (or follow directions on flatbread packaging).

2. In a small bowl, combine the Greek yogurt, mayonnaise, and ranch seasoning. Stir until well combined.

3. Use a rubber spatula or the back of a spoon to spread the ranch sauce evenly over the flatbread, leaving about a ½-inch (27 cm) bare around the sides for the crust. Top the sauce with ½ cup (77 g) of pickles. Sprinkle the mozzarella and the provolone on top. Evenly spread the shredded chicken over the cheese. Top with the remaining ½ cup (77 g) pickles and dill.

4. Bake directly on a rack in the oven for 5 to 7 minutes for a crispy crust or bake on a sheet pan for 5 to 9 minutes for a softer crust. Drizzle with hot honey.

5. Cut into squares and enjoy!

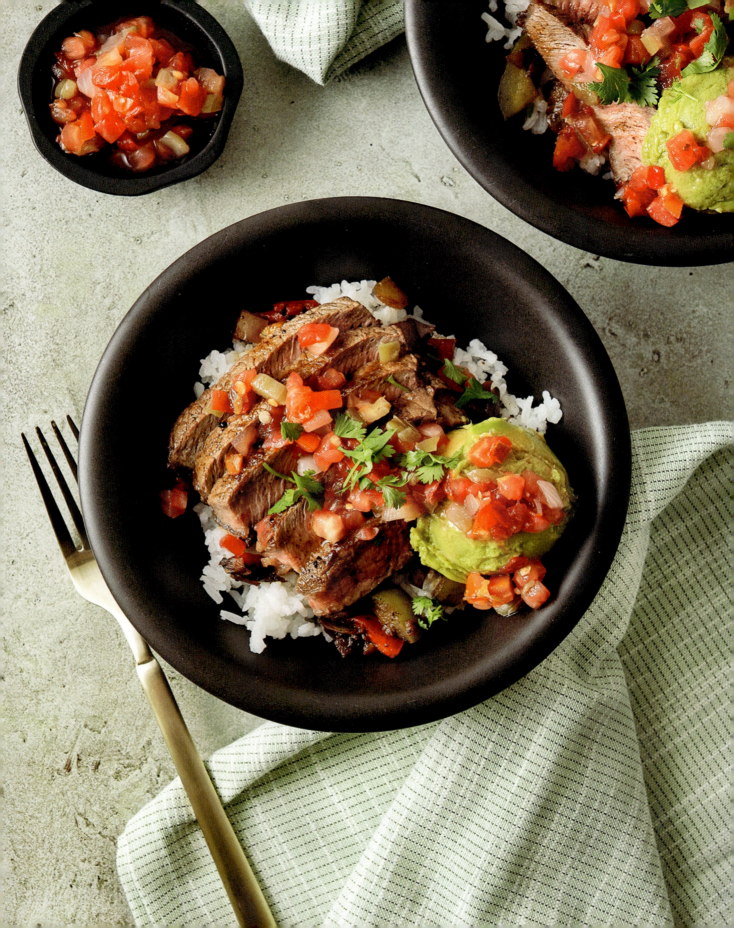

Steak or Shrimp Fajita Bowl

I love a good Chipotle bowl, especially when I save some money making my own version at home. Shortcuts in this recipe include using a frozen fajita veggie blend, 90-second rice, and pre-made fajita spice blend.

Yield: 2 servings

Ingredients

- ½ pound (227 g) sirloin steak or ½ pound (227 g) deveined shrimp
- 2 tablespoons (6 g) low-sodium fajita spice blend, divided
- 2 teaspoons red wine vinegar, divided
- 3 tablespoons (45 ml) olive oil, divided
- 1 cup (150 g) frozen fajita veggie blend, defrosted
- 90-second packet of rice
- 2 2-ounce (56 g) Guacamole single serve cups
- 4 tablespoons (60 ml) pico de gallo, divided

You Will Need

- Paper towel
- Large mixing bowl
- Measuring spoons
- Medium nonstick skillet
- Tongs
- Cutting board
- Sheet pan
- Cooking spray

Instructions

If Making Steak:

1. Pat steak dry with paper towel and place in a large mixing bowl. Add 1 tablespoon (3 g) fajita spice blend, 1 tablespoon (15 ml) olive oil, 1 teaspoon red wine vinegar, and salt and pepper to taste to the bowl and toss steak in the seasonings until it is well-coated.

2. Add 1 tablespoon (15 ml) olive oil to a medium nonstick skillet over medium-high heat. When oil is slightly shimmering add the steak and cook for 3 to 4 minutes per side for a medium-rare steak (about 130ºF to 135ºF [54ºC to 57ºC]; cook longer for desired doneness). Transfer to a cutting board and let cool for at least 5 minutes before slicing into ½-inch (1 cm) thick slices against the grain.

If Making Shrimp:

1. Pat shrimp dry with a paper towel. In a mixing bowl, combine the shrimp, 1 tablespoon (3 g) fajita spice blend, 1 tablespoon (15 ml) olive oil, and salt and pepper to taste. Toss until shrimp are well-coated.

2. Add 1 tablespoon (15 ml) olive oil to a medium nonstick skillet and place over medium heat. When oil is slightly shimmering add shrimp and cook for 2 to 3 minutes per side. Transfer to clean cutting board.

Finish Fajitas:

1. Return medium nonstick skillet to the stove. Add 1 tablespoon (15 ml) olive oil and the frozen fajita veggie blend and cook, stirring often until the veggies are soft and starting to char, about 5 to 7 minutes. Remove the pan from the heat.

2. Microwave the rice according to package directions. Add half of the rice, the steak or shrimp, veggies, 1 single-serve cup of guacamole and 2 tablespoons (30 ml) of pico de gallo to a bowl. Enjoy!

Six-Ingredient Chicken and Veggie Stir-Fry

This is one of my go-to heat and eat meals. It's a great example of how you can utilize processed foods to make assembling a meal at home more accessible for the ADHD brain. I like to use microwave rice pouches because there are fewer dishes. If you want to cook your own rice, I highly recommend a rice cooker, so you don't have to worry about burning the rice if you forget about it. It also keeps the rice warm.

Yield: 2 servings

Ingredients

- 2 tablespoons (30 ml) sesame oil
- 1 frozen ginger cube or 1 teaspoon raw ginger
- 2 cups (330 g) frozen stir-fry veggie mix
- 6 ounces (170 g) frozen grilled diced chicken
- 1 pouch 90-second rice
- 2 ounces (56 g) store-bought stir-fry sauce

You Will Need

- Measuring spoons
- Wok or large nonstick pan
- Spatula
- ¼- and 1-cup measuring cups

Instructions

1. Heat sesame oil in a wok or large nonstick pan over medium-high heat. Once the oil is heated and shimmering add the ginger and stir-fry veggie mix to the wok and cook for 3 to 4 minutes, stirring occasionally. Reduce heat to medium. Add the chicken to the wok with the veggies. Continue cooking for another 3 to 5 minutes, or until the chicken is heated through.

2. While the veggies and chicken cook, heat the microwave rice according to the directions on the pouch.

3. Add the stir-fry sauce to the wok and toss until well combined. Divide rice, the chicken, and the veggies into two bowls. Enjoy!

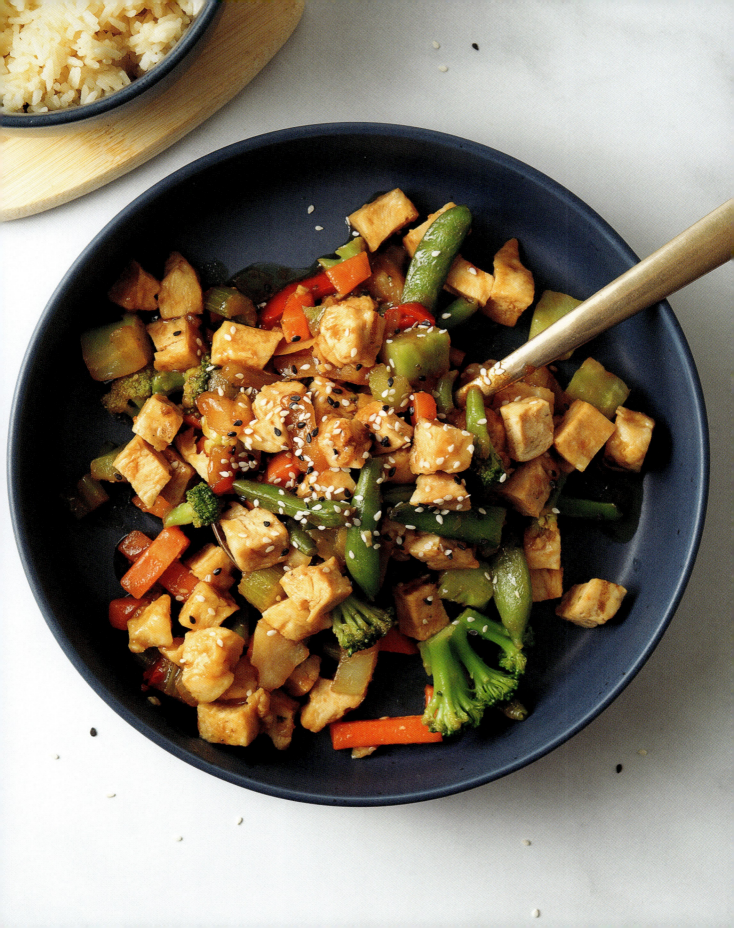

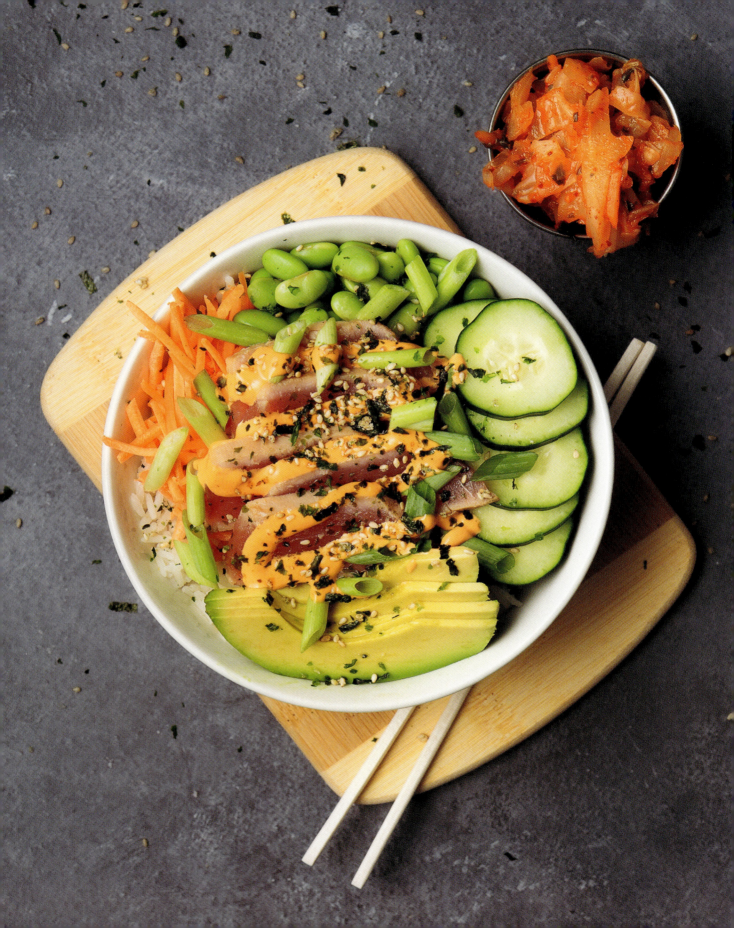

Teriyaki Tuna Bowl

I love poke bowls, and it's easier than you'd think to make your own poke style bowl at home. Tuna is an excellent source of EPA and DHA, which are the types of omega-3s that are important for ADHD brains. This bowl uses a store-bought teriyaki sauce to save time (I prefer the Soyaki sauce from Trader Joe's), but feel free to make your own sauce if you're feeling fancy. You can and should also switch up the toppings to meet your preferences.

Yield: 2 bowls

Ingredients

- 2 [4-ounce (114 g)], 1-inch (2.5 cm) thick Ahi tuna steaks
- ⅓ cup (79 ml) store-bought Teriyaki sauce
- 1 tablespoon (15 ml) canola oil
- 1 90-second rice packet
- 1 cup (155 g) frozen edamame, thawed
- ½ cup (55 g) shredded carrots
- 1 mini cucumber, sliced
- 1 medium avocado (about 150 g), sliced
- 2 green onions, thinly sliced
- 1 teaspoon sesame seeds, divided
- 2 tablespoons (28 g) spicy mayo
- Sriracha to taste (optional)

Additional optional toppings: Store-bought seaweed salad, kimchi, pickled radishes, seaweed, furikake seasoning, mango, or wasabi

You Will Need

- Large Ziploc bag
- ⅓ and ½-cup measuring cups
- Cutting board
- Utility knife
- Medium nonstick pan
- Measurement spoons
- Tongs

Instructions

1. Place tuna steaks in a Ziploc bag and add teriyaki sauce to coat. Transfer the bag to the fridge to marinate for 10 to 15 minutes while you prep the veggies.

2. Heat a medium nonstick pan over medium-high until hot. Add 1 tablespoon (15 ml) canola oil to the pan. Sear the tuna on both sides to your desired doneness: 30 seconds for rare, 1 to 1½ minutes for medium-rare, 2 to 2½ minutes for medium-well to well. Once cooked, transfer the steaks to a cutting board and slice immediately into ½-inch-thick (2.5-cm) slices.

3. Microwave rice according to package directions. Divide heated rice into two bowls. Add sliced tuna steak, edamame, carrots, cucumber, avocado, and green onions to the rice bowl. Top with a sprinkle of sesame seeds, drizzle of spicy mayo, and optional Sriracha for more heat. Enjoy!

NOTES: If you let the tuna steaks rest before slicing, they will continue to cook, so don't hesitate!

Sheet Pan Gnocchi and Veggies

This is one of my favorite vegetarian sheet pan meals. I really like how the gnocchi gets a little crispy in the oven, so there's more crunch than with regular gnocchi. I save a couple steps by buying pre-chopped peppers and butternut squash.

Yield: 2 servings

Ingredients

- 1 [1 pound (453 g)] package of uncooked gnocchi
- 1 medium red bell pepper, chopped
- 1 pint cherry tomatoes
- ½ red onion, chopped
- 1 bag cubed butternut squash
- 4 tablespoons (60 ml) olive oil
- 2 teaspoons jarred minced garlic
- 1 teaspoon Italian seasoning
- Salt and pepper to taste
- ¼ cup (22 g) Parmesan cheese, for topping

You Will Need

- Sheet pan
- Silicone baking mat or aluminum foil
- Cooking spray
- Knife
- Cutting board
- Measuring spoons
- ¼-cup measuring cup

Instructions

1. Preheat oven to 425°F (218°C). Line sheet pan with silicone baking mat or aluminum foil and spray with cooking spray.

2. Spread gnocchi, red bell pepper, cherry tomatoes, red onion, and butternut squash on the sheet pan. Drizzle the olive oil over the gnocchi and veggies. Add the minced garlic, Italian seasoning, and salt and pepper to the sheet pan. Toss well to coat the gnocchi and veggies with the oil and seasonings.

3. Place the sheet pan in the oven. Bake for 25 to 30 minutes and toss midway through roasting. The tomatoes should be bursting and the veggies should be soft and slightly browned.

4. Serve gnocchi and veggies in a bowl topped with parmesan cheese and enjoy!

Chicken Tender Wrap

This is a twist on the McDonald's Snack Wrap. I swapped the American cheese for pepper-jack and the ranch dressing for avocado ranch dressing. I prefer using a low-carb wrap because they are higher in fiber, which helps keep me full for longer. You can use any chicken tenders you like and save yourself an extra step by buying prechopped lettuce.

Yield: 1 wrap

Ingredients

- 2 frozen chicken tenders
- 1 low-carb street taco-sized tortilla
- 2 tablespoons (30 ml) store-bought avocado ranch dressing
- 1 slice pepper jack cheese
- 1 handful shredded lettuce
- 4 pickled jalapeño slices

You Will Need

- Air Fryer
- Tongs
- Plate

Instructions

1. Cook chicken tenders in air fryer according to package directions.

2. Lay tortilla on a plate. Drizzle ranch on the tortilla. Lay the chicken tenders vertically in the center of the tortilla. Add the cheese, lettuce, and pickles.

3. Fold the bottom of tortilla in toward the ends of the chicken tenders to create the bottom of the wrap. Then, fold each of the sides of the tortilla in to cover the chicken tenders and form a wrap.

Shrimp Tostadas

Shrimp is a great protein for ADHDers, because it is an excellent source of magnesium and zinc, which are two minerals that many ADHDers probably don't eat enough of. One cool part of this recipe is that you don't cook the shrimp with heat. Instead, the acid from the lime juice marinade will denature or breakdown the proteins. I make this for dinner and have the leftovers the next day for an easy lunch, that only requires me to assemble the tostadas.

Yield: 2 servings

Ingredients

- 1 pound (453 g) fresh shrimp, peeled and deveined
- 1 11-ounce (331 g) can fiesta-style corn, drained
- 1 10-ounce (284 g) container store-bought pico de gallo
- 1 medium avocado, diced
- ¼ cup (13 g) red onion, diced
- 1 7-ounce (198 g) can diced green chiles (optional)
- 2 tablespoon (30 ml) lime juice
- 2 tablespoons (30 ml) lemon juice
- 1 tablespoon (4 g) fresh cilantro, chopped
- Salt to taste
- 6 corn tortillas
- Cooking spray
- ¼ cup (60 g) fresh cotija cheese

You Will Need

- Knife
- Cutting board
- Medium bowl
- ¼-cup measuring cup
- Measuring spoons
- Air fryer
- Cooking spray
- Can opener

Instructions

1. Chop shrimp into small pieces and add to a medium bowl. Add the fiesta corn, pico de gallo, avocado, red onion, green chiles, lime juice, lemon juice, and cilantro to the bowl and mix to combine. Salt to taste and set the bowl aside to let marinate.

2. Spray both sides of each tortilla with cooking spray.

3. Lay one or two tortillas in the air-fryer basket. If you add more than one tortilla, make sure they do not overlap. You may have to put a heat-safe cup on top of the tortillas to prevent air pockets from forming. Set the air fryer to 300°F (149°C) and cook for about 6 minutes, or until the tortillas are crispy and golden brown in color. Repeat with the rest of the tortillas.

4. Divide the tortillas between two plates. Top each tortilla with ⅙ of the shrimp mixture and garnish with a sprinkle of cotija cheese.

Cheesy Chicken Nachos

Nachos are fun and easy to customize to fit your sensory preferences. I use rotisserie chicken in this recipe, but you can use leftover taco meat from the Walking "Tacos" (page 142) or another protein of your choice. I've also added beans for some extra fiber and protein. My shortcuts for this recipe are to buy prechopped tomatoes, red onion, and pickled jalapeños to save some steps.

Yield: 2 servings

Ingredients

- 1 cup (135 g) shredded rotisserie chicken
- ¾ cup (194 g) salsa, divided
- 3 to 4 cups (78 to 104 g) tortilla chips
- ½ cup (90 g) low-sodium black beans, rinsed and drained
- ¼ cup (50 g) diced tomatoes
- ¼ cup (13 g) diced red onion
- 1 to 2 tablespoons (15 to 30 g) diced jalapeños
- 1 cup (100 g) shredded Mexican cheese
- ¼ cup (60 g) guacamole
- ¼ cup (50 g) sour cream or nonfat Greek yogurt

You Will Need

- Microwave safe bowl
- Air Fryer
- Cooking spray
- Can opener
- 1-cup and ¼-cup measuring cups
- Measuring spoons

Instructions

1. Place shredded chicken in microwave safe bowl. Microwave for 1 to 2 minutes to warm up chicken. Add ½ cup (129 g) of salsa to the bowl. Toss to coat the chicken well with the salsa.

2. Spray air fryer basket with cooking spray. Add tortilla chips to the air fryer basket, arranging them as evenly as possible. Next, layer the chicken, black beans, tomatoes, red onion, and jalapeños.

3. Place the basket in the air fryer and cook at 400°F (204ºC) for 6 to 8 minutes. Transfer to plates and top with cheese, guacamole, and sour cream or nonfat Greek yogurt. Enjoy!

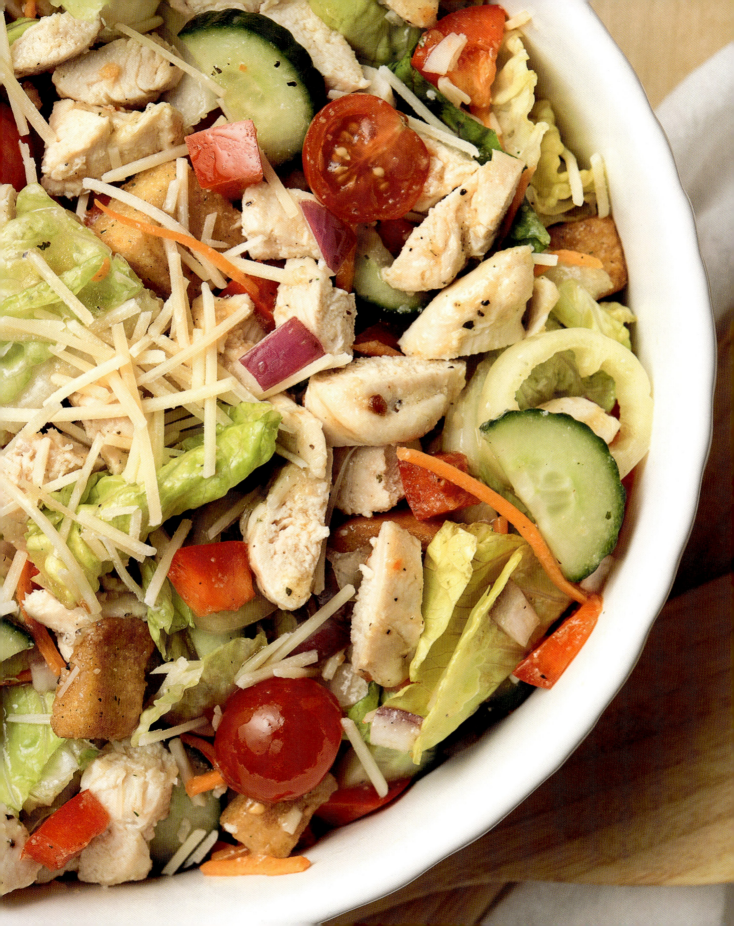

Loaded Veggie Salad with Grilled Chicken

My partner Tim and I like to use the air fryer to batch cook chicken for the week and this is one of our go-to ways to use the chicken. The star of this salad is Tim's flavorful salad dressing, which also doubles as the marinade for the chicken. When we make this salad, we chop all the veggies and whatever we don't use for the salad we store in separate containers. That way we can keep making quick salads or use the veggies in other dishes throughout the week. You can add whatever veggies you like to this salad and even buy pre-cut veggies to make it easier.

Yield: 3 to 4 servings

Ingredients

- ¼ cup (59 ml) red wine vinegar
- 3 tablespoons (45 ml) water
- 1 packet Italian dressing mix
- ½ cup (118 ml) olive oil
- 1 pound (454 g) chicken tenderloins
- 1 head romaine lettuce, chopped
- ½ cup (110 ml) shredded carrots
- ⅓ cup (38 g) red onion, chopped
- ½ cup (90 g) red bell pepper, chopped
- ½ cup (75 g) cucumber, halved
- 1 cup (149 g) cherry tomatoes, halved
- ¼ cup (31 g) banana peppers, sliced
- 1 cup (42 g) croutons
- ¼ cup (25 g) shredded parmesan cheese (optional)

You Will Need

- 32-ounce (907 g) airtight container for dressing
- ¼-, ⅓-, and ½-cup measuring cups
- Measuring spoons
- Paper towel
- Medium bowl
- Air fryer
- Food thermometer
- Cutting board
- Knife
- Large salad bowl

Instructions

To Make the Salad Dressing/Marinade:

1. Pour vinegar and water into an airtight container. Add packet of Italian dressing mix to container. Cover and shake vigorously to combine. Remove the lid and add olive oil. Cover and shake again. Makes 1 cup (236 ml).

To Make the Loaded Veggie Salad:

1. Pat chicken dry with paper towel and place in a medium bowl. Add ½ cup (118 ml) of marinade to the bowl and toss until chicken is well coated. Set chicken in fridge to marinate for at least minutes.

2. Place chicken in the air fryer basket and cook at 400°F (204°C) for 15 to 18 minutes, or until chicken is cooked to internal temperature of 165°F (74°C).

3. While chicken cooks, cut up the veggies and add them to a large salad bowl. Add croutons and parmesan to the salad bowl. Pour ½ cup (118 ml) of the salad dressing into the bowl and toss to combine. Divide the salad evenly between the bowls.

4. After chicken is cooked, cut it into bite sized pieces. Top bowls with chicken. Enjoy!

Teriyaki Salmon Burgers

These burgers are tangy and delicious and inspired by the teriyaki chicken burgers I ate growing up. Save yourself a step in this recipe by using frozen sweet potato fries. If you can, add the burgers, pineapple, and sweet potato fries to the air fryer basket at the same time. If not, do the burger and pineapple and then the fries.

Yield: 2 servings

Ingredients

- 1 5-ounce (142 g) can salmon
- ¼ cup (38 g) panko breadcrumbs
- ¼ cup (37 g) red bell pepper, diced
- ¼ cup (26 g) green onions, diced
- 2 teaspoons Sriracha, divided
- 1 large egg
- 2 frozen ginger cubes, thawed
- 2 tablespoons (30 ml) teriyaki sauce
- 1 tablespoon (9 g) sesame seeds
- 2 teaspoons sesame oil
- 1 teaspoon garlic powder
- Salt and pepper to taste
- 2 canned pineapple rings
- 1 sweet potato, cut into ¼-inch (6 mm) slices
- 2 teaspoons olive oil
- 2 hamburger buns
- ¼ red onion, sliced
- 1 teaspoon Sriracha
- 2 tablespoons (28 g) mayo

You Will Need

- 2 medium bowls
- Can opener
- Knife
- Cutting board
- ¼-cup measuring cup
- Measuring spoons
- Rubber spatula
- Cooking spray
- Air fryer
- Small bowl

Instructions

1. In a medium bowl, add canned salmon, panko, red bell pepper, green onion, 1 teaspoon Sriracha, egg, ginger cubes, teriyaki sauce, sesame seeds, sesame oil, garlic powder, and salt and pepper to taste. Use your hands or a spatula to combine everything, then divide and form the mixture into 2 patties.

2. Spray air fryer basket with cooking spray. Add the salmon patties and pineapple rings side by side in the basket. Cook at 400°F (204°C) for 5 minutes. Flip the patties and cook for an additional 5 minutes.

3. While the burgers cook, add sweet potatoes, olive oil, and salt and pepper to a medium bowl. Toss to coat the sweet potatoes.

4. After the burgers and pineapple are done cooking, remove them from the basket and cover to keep warm. Spray empty basket with cooking spray and add the sweet potato fries to basket. Cook at 400°F (204°C) for about 10 minutes, tossing halfway through.

5. While fries are cooking, combine 1 teaspoon Sriracha and 2 tablespoons (28 g) mayo in a small bowl to make a spicy mayo.

6. When the fries are done, you may want to add burgers back to air fryer for 2 to 3 minutes to heat them up. Open buns and spread half of spicy mayo on one side of each burger bun. Layer the salmon burger, pineapple, and red onion slices on the bottom of piece of the bun. Place the top half of bun on top. Serve with sweet potato fries.

InstantPot Vegetarian chili

I always look forward to a big bowl of chili on a cool fall day. Chili is a hearty, high-fiber meal. I love it because it's a dump and heat dish that you can batch cook to freeze for later or eat throughout the week. I also enjoy switching up the toppings to add variety.

Yield: 6 to 8 servings

Ingredients

- 1 medium yellow onion, finely chopped
- 1 14.5-ounce (411 g) can red kidney beans, drained and rinsed
- 1 14.5-ounce (411 g) can black beans, drained and rinsed
- 1 14.5-ounce (411 g) can pinto beans, drained and rinsed
- 1 14.5-ounce (411 g) can whole peeled tomatoes
- 1 14.5-ounce (411 g) can fire roasted tomatoes with garlic
- 1 14.5-ounce (411 g) can diced tomatoes with green chilies
- 2 teaspoons jarred minced garlic (add more if you'd like)
- 1 teaspoon smoked paprika
- 1 tablespoon (8 g) chili powder
- 1 teaspoon cumin
- Salt and pepper to taste

Optional toppings: shredded Monterey Jack cheese, sour cream, sliced jalapeño peppers

You Will Need

- InstantPot or slow cooker (see note)
- Can opener
- Spoon
- Plastic colander
- Measuring spoons

Instructions

1. Add all of the ingredients to the InstantPot (see note if using a slow cooker). Stir the mixture to combine.

2. Seal the lid on the InstantPot and set it to the soup setting. Release pressure when timer goes off or let it depressurize on its own.

3. Remove the lid and stir to make sure everything is nicely mixed. Serve in a bowl with your favorite toppings.

Note: If using a slow cooker, simply dump everything in the slow cooker and cook on low for about 6 hours.

Kitchen Sink Veggie Soup

Veggie soup is a great way to get your veggies in! The chickpeas in this recipe add some protein.

Yield: 4 servings

Ingredients

- 1 14.5-ounce (411 g) can chickpeas
- 8 cups (1.8 L) low-sodium vegetable broth
- 1 12-ounce (340 g) bag frozen mirepoix blend (celery, onion, carrots)
- 1 10-ounce (283 g) bag frozen yellow corn
- 2 14.5-ounce (411 g) cans of stewed tomatoes
- 1 tablespoon (14 g) garlic, minced
- 2 tablespoons (7 g) Italian seasoning
- Salt and pepper to taste

You Will Need

- Can opener
- Liquid measuring cup
- Measuring spoons
- InstantPot or slow cooker (see note)
- Spoon

Instructions

1. Add all of the ingredients to the InstantPot (see note if using a slow cooker) and stir to combine.

2. Seal the lid on InstantPot and set it to the soup setting.

3. Release pressure when timer goes off or let it depressurize on its own. Remove lid and stir. Serve in a bowl. Enjoy!

Note: If using a slow cooker, simply dump everything into the slow cooker and cook on low for about 6 hours.

Falafel Hummus Platter

This is fun meal is a variation of ADHD charcuterie that you can eat with your hands. I really like dips so I try to find ways that I can incorporate them into my meals. Buy frozen premade falafel to save a few steps!

Yield: 3 servings

Ingredients

- 1 10.5-ounce (288 g) bag frozen premade falafel
- 3 pitas, cut into triangles
- 3 mini cucumbers, sliced
- 8 mini peppers
- 2 cups (284 g) baby carrots
- ½ cup (125 g) hummus of your choice and/or tzatziki

You Will Need

- Baking sheet
- Cooking spray
- Spatula
- Cutting board
- Knife

Instructions

1. Preheat oven to 350°F (177°C). Spray baking sheet with cooking spray. Arrange falafel on a baking sheet and bake for 10 minutes.

2. Use a spatula to flip the falafel and cook for an additional 8 to 10 minutes until thoroughly heated.

3. While the falafel is baking, divide the veggies and dips onto three plates.

4. Remove the falafel from the oven and allow it to cool for a few minutes. Divide the falafel evenly between three plates and serve with vegetables and hummus or tzatziki. Enjoy!

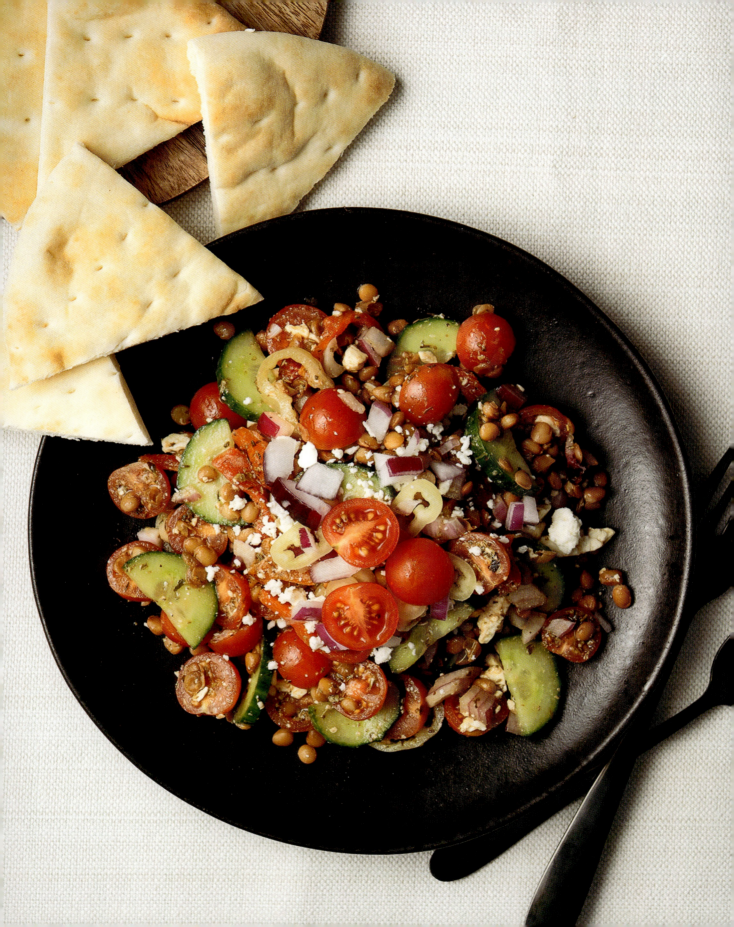

Greek-Style Lentil Salad

This is technically a no-heat recipe if you buy lentils that are precooked or canned. Lentils are an underrated legume that provide 18 g protein and 16 g fiber in a single one-cup serving! They're also a great source of iron, which many ADHDers don't get enough of. We should all eat more lentils.

This is a dish that gets better as the flavors marinate, so don't skip the refrigeration time. You can easily make this completely vegan by leaving out the feta or swapping it for vegan cheese.

Yield: 5 servings

Ingredients

- ½ medium cucumber, sliced and halved
- ½ cup (240 g) roasted red pepper, roughly chopped
- ½ cup (58 g) red onion, chopped
- ¼ cup (31 g) banana peppers, sliced
- 1 pint (340 g) cherry tomatoes, halved
- ½ cup (123 g) feta cheese crumbles
- 1 1-pound (456 g) package steamed ready-to-eat lentils
- 1 tablespoon (4 g) Italian seasoning
- 2 tablespoons (30 ml) olive oil
- 2 tablespoons (30 ml) balsamic vinegar
- 1 tablespoon (15 ml) lemon juice
- Salt and pepper to taste

You Will Need

- Large mixing bowl
- Knife
- Cutting board
- ¼- and ½-cup measuring cups
- Measuring spoons
- Rubber spatula
- Beeswax or plastic wrap

Instructions

1. Add all ingredients to a large mixing bowl and toss to combine. Cover with beeswax or plastic wrap and refrigerate for at least an hour to let the flavors meld.

2. Once ready, serve in a bowl and enjoy!

3. Store in an airtight container for up to 5 days.

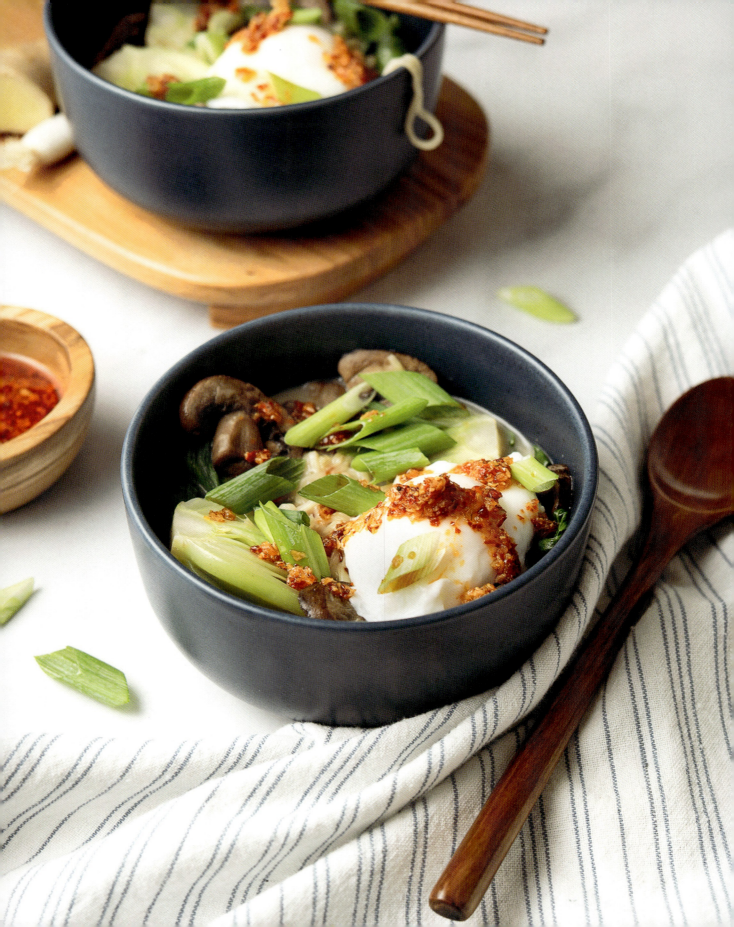

Ramen Glow-up

I love a bowl of instant ramen on its own, especially when I'm sick or don't have much of an appetite, but if I want ramen to fill me up, I gotta add some extra toppings. These are the toppings I like to add to my ramen when I need to give it a bit of a glow-up, but I invite you to tap into your creative side and add what you enjoy.

Yield: 1 to 2 servings

Ingredients

- 2 teaspoons sesame oil
- 1 teaspoon minced ginger
- 1 teaspoon minced garlic
- ½ cup (35 g) sliced baby bella mushrooms
- 1 cup (237 ml) miso broth
- 1 cup (237 ml) water
- 1 instant ramen package (noodles only—discard the seasoning packet)
- 2 bunches baby bok choy, halved lengthwise
- 2 large eggs
- 1 green onion, thinly sliced diagonally
- Drizzle of chili crunch oil

You Will Need

- Small pot
- Measuring spoons
- ½-cup measuring cup
- Liquid measuring cup
- Knife
- Cutting board

Instructions

1. Place a small pot over medium-high heat. Add the oil, ginger, and garlic and cook until fragrant, about 1 minute. Add mushrooms to the pot and sauté for 2 more minutes, or until softened. Create your ramen broth by adding the miso broth and water to the pot and bringing it to a boil.

2. Add instant ramen noodles to the broth and boil for about 4 minutes. Stir in bok choy.

3. Turn heat to low and crack eggs directly into the broth. Let eggs cook undisturbed for seven minutes or until the egg whites are cooked and the yolks are jammy.

4. Pour the ramen into a bowl for one large serving or divide between two bowls for two smaller servings. Garnish with sliced green onion and a drizzle of chili crunch oil. Enjoy!

Note: I buy frozen minced ginger and garlic cubes to save time. Each cube is 1 teaspoon. If using frozen garlic and ginger in this recipe, follow the directions as listed and simply cook until thawed.

Chicken and Broccoli Mac and Cheese

As a kid, I enjoyed all three of these foods at meals separately, now I enjoy serving them together in a bowl. I like to use either Goodles or Banza boxed cheddar elbows because they have more protein and fiber than traditional mac and cheese. Broccoli is an excellent source of vitamin C, which plays a role in dopamine production, so it's a great veggie for ADHDers to incorporate into their meals.

Yield: 2 servings

Ingredients

- 1 box mac and cheese
- ¼ cup (59 ml) low-fat milk
- 2 tablespoons (28 g) butter
- 6 ounces (168 g) frozen precooked grilled chicken strips
- 2 cups (368 g) frozen broccoli florets

You Will Need

- Medium pot
- Liquid measuring cup
- Measuring spoons
- ¼-cup measuring cup
- Colander
- Mixing spoon
- Medium nonstick pan
- Cooking spray
- Spatula or tongs

Instructions

1. In a medium pot, cook mac and cheese according to the directions on the box.

2. Heat a medium, nonstick pan over medium-high heat. Spray the pan with cooking spray. Add chicken and broccoli and cover with a lid. Stir occasionally and cook until heated.

3. Divide mac and cheese into two bowls, top with chicken and broccoli, and enjoy!

Sausage and Veggie Pasta

If you want a more nutrient-dense, delicious pasta recipe, this is it! This pasta dish is great because it's high in fiber and protein, which are the two nutrients I recommend focusing on for gentle nutrition. I use frozen veggies so the only prep is chopping the chicken sausage.

Yield: 4 servings

Ingredients

- 2 cups (50 g) penne protein pasta
- 4 tablespoons (60 ml) avocado oil, divided
- 4 Italian style chicken sausages, cut into ¼-inch (6 mm) coins
- 1 [1-pound (453 g)] bag frozen veggie blend (see note)
- 2 teaspoons jarred minced garlic
- ⅔ cup (158 ml) heavy cream
- ¼ cup (28 g) freshly grated parmesan (optional)
- Salt and pepper to taste

You Will Need

- Medium pot
- Liquid measuring cup
- Colander
- Measuring spoons
- Large skillet
- Spatula
- Slotted spoon
- ¼-cup and ⅓-cup measuring cups

Instructions

1. Bring a medium pot of salted water to a boil. Add the pasta and cook until al dente. Reserve ⅓ cup (79 ml) of pasta water before draining. Return the pasta to the pot and toss with 2 tablespoons (30 ml) avocado oil.

2. In a large skillet, add 2 tablespoons (30 ml) avocado oil and place over medium-high heat. Add chicken sausage to the skillet and cook until both sides of the sausage are browned. Transfer the chicken sausage to the pot with the pasta using a slotted spoon.

3. Add veggie blend to the skillet. Season with salt and pepper to taste. Sauté the veggies until tender. Add the pasta and chicken sausages to the skillet with the veggies. Add minced garlic and heavy cream, stir and bring the liquid to a boil. Cook until the cream has thickened. Adjust seasonings if needed.

4. Serve in a bowl topped with fresh grated parmesan cheese. Store the reserved pasta water in an airtight container in the fridge, and add to leftovers before reheating to loosen the sauce.

Note: I like to use a Mediterranean veggie blend for this recipe, so it has zucchini, squash, carrots, green beans, bell peppers, and onions.

Muffin Pan Chicken Pot Pies

Chicken pot pies are a classic comfort food. This is a great way to use rotisserie chicken, and the leftovers freeze beautifully so you can save what you don't eat for a later meal.

Yield: 12 pot pies

Ingredients

- 1 [12-ounce (340 g)] bag frozen mirepoix blend (celery, onion, carrots), defrosted
- ½ cup (80 g) frozen peas, defrosted
- 1 cup (135 g) shredded rotisserie chicken
- About ¾ of a 10.5-ounce (233 ml) can 98% fat-free condensed cream of chicken soup
- ¼ teaspoon Italian seasoning
- ½ teaspoon garlic powder
- Salt and pepper to taste
- Flour for dusting
- 1 [17.3-ounce (490 g)] package frozen puff pastry sheets, thawed
- 1 large egg

You Will Need

- Cooking spray
- 12-count muffin pan
- Medium mixing bowl
- Mixing spoon
- Rolling pin
- Small bowl
- Fork
- Brush

Instructions

1. Preheat oven to 425°F (218°C).

2. In a medium bowl, add the mirepoix, peas, chicken, condensed soup, Italian seasoning, and garlic powder. Mix with a spoon to combine. Season with salt and pepper.

3. Use cooking spray to grease a 12-cup muffin pan. Lightly dust a clean surface with flour. Roll 1 puff pastry sheet onto the lightly dusted surface to get it out of its folded shape. Cut puff pastry into 6 even squares. Repeat with the other puff pastry sheet.

4. Press a square of puff pastry into each of the muffin cups in the prepared pan, arranging so they fully line the cup and form a well. (The sides and corners of the squares will spill over the sides of the muffin cups). Add 4 tablespoons (34 g) of the pot pie mixture to each cup. Fold the corners of the puff pastry over the mixture and pinch them together so the mixture is sealed within the puff pastry.

5. Create an egg wash by beating an egg and 1 tablespoon (15 ml) water in a small bowl. Brush the tops of the puff pastry with egg wash.

6. Place muffin pan in the oven and cook for 25 to 28 minutes, or until the crust is crispy and a warm golden color. Let cool for about 5 minutes before removing from the pan. Serve on a plate. Store any leftover pot pies in an airtight container for up to 5 days.

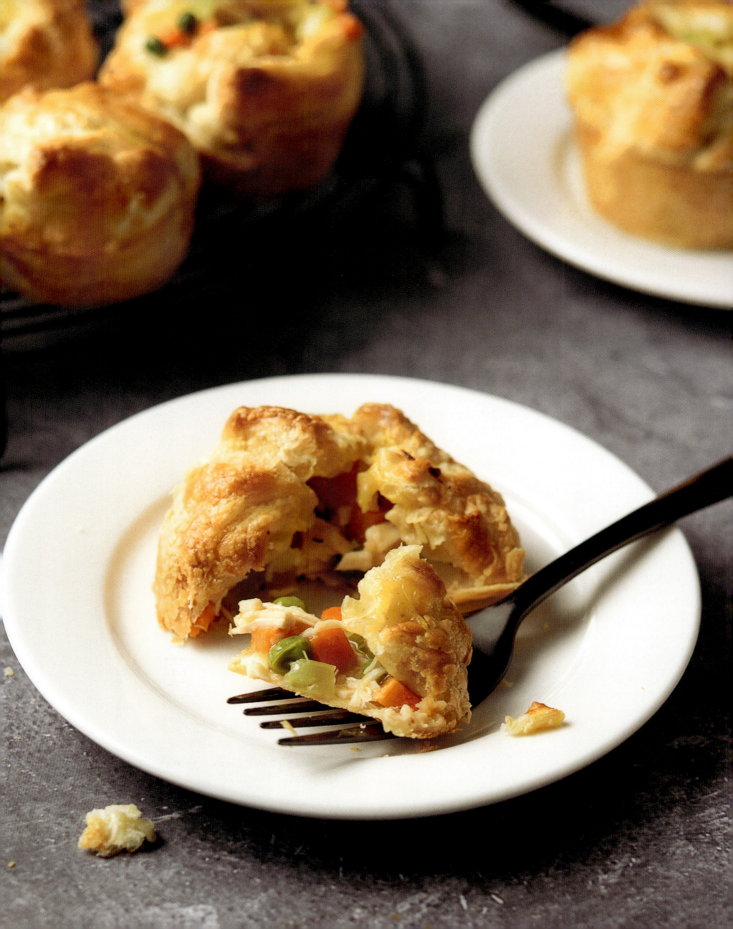

Cheeseburger Casserole

Casseroles are great for families or if you want to batch cook one thing to eat throughout the week. This is a fancier version of the Hamburger Helper Cheeseburger Macaroni. I didn't grow up on Hamburger Helper, but I know a lot of people did, so this one's for you!

Yield: 3 to 5 servings

Ingredients

- 6 ounces (170g) dried elbow macaroni pasta
- 1 pound (454 g) lean ground beef
- 2 teaspoons Italian seasoning, divided
- ½ teaspoon salt
- ½ teaspoon pepper
- ¼ teaspoon dry mustard
- ½ teaspoon paprika
- ¼ teaspoon cayenne pepper
- 1 teaspoon butter
- ½ cup (58 g) chopped yellow onion
- 1 tablespoon (10 g) jarred minced garlic
- 2 tablespoons (28 g) tomato paste
- 1¼ cups (296 ml) heavy cream
- ¼ cup (59 ml) water
- 1 cup (100 g) shredded cheddar cheese, divided
- 1 cup (100 g) Colby jack cheese, divided

You Will Need

- Large pot
- Colander
- Large skillet
- Slotted spoon
- Measuring spoons
- ½-cup and 1-cup measuring cups
- Liquid measuring cup
- 8" x 8" (20 x 20 cm) pan
- Cooking spray
- Serving spoon

Instructions

1. Preheat the oven to 400°F (204°C).

2. Bring a large pot of salted water to a boil. Add the pasta and cook for 9 to 11 minutes uncovered and stir occasionally. Once pasta is mostly cooked through, drain in a colander and set aside.

3. Place a large skillet on medium heat. Add the ground beef, onion, 1 teaspoon Italian seasoning, salt, pepper, dry mustard, paprika, and cayenne pepper. Cook for about 5 minutes or until browned, breaking up the ground beef with a wooden spoon. Add the pasta, butter, garlic, tomato paste, heavy cream, water, and remaining Italian seasoning to the skillet. Stir well to combine.

4. Transfer the mixture to an 8" x 8" (20 x 20 cm) ungreased casserole dish. Cover with aluminum foil and bake in the oven for about minutes. Remove from the oven. Sprinkle ¾ cup (25 g) shredded cheddar cheese and ¾ cup (25 g) shredded Colby jack cheese over the casserole. Top with remaining shredded cheeses.

5. Return casserole to the oven uncovered and bake for additional 15 minutes or until the cheese is browned and bubbly. Serve casserole on plates and enjoy!

6. Store in an airtight container in the refrigerator for up to 3 days or freeze for up to 3 months.

Energy Balls—3 Ways

Fun and kid-friendly, these are a great snack option if you want to pack some solid nutrition into just a couple of bites.

Yield: 10 to 15 balls

Ingredients

Energy Ball Base
- ½ cup (45 g) old fashioned oats
- 2 tablespoons (32 g) creamy peanut butter (see note)
- 2 tablespoons (20 g) chia seeds
- 3 tablespoons (45 ml) sweetener of choice, such as honey
- ½ teaspoon vanilla extract
- Dash of flakey sea salt

Peanut Butter Dark Chocolate Balls
- 2 tablespoons (28 g) peanut butter chips
- 2 tablespoons (28 g) dark chocolate chips

Strawberry Shortcake Balls
- 2 tablespoons (28 g) vanilla protein powder
- ⅓ cup (7 g) crushed freeze dried strawberries
- 2 teaspoons strawberry jam (optional)

"Kitchen Sink" Balls
- 2 tablespoons (10 g) mini M&Ms
- 2 tablespoons (5 g) pretzels, chopped
- 2 tablespoons (28 g) chopped walnuts

You Will Need
- Medium mixing bowl
- ⅓-cup and ½-cup measuring cups
- Measuring spoons
- Spatula
- Plastic wrap

Instructions

1. In a medium bowl, add all the ingredients from the base recipe plus the ingredients from whichever variation you are making. Use a rubber spatula to combine the ingredients. Cover the mixture with plastic wrap and refrigerate for at least 2 hours or until the mixture is chilled.

2. Remove the bowl from the fridge and use your hands to form the mixture into 10 to 15 [1-inch (2.5 cm)] balls. Store in an airtight container or freeze for up to 3 months.

Note: Swap peanut butter for sunflower butter if you have a nut allergy.

Smoked Salmon Dip

The next few recipes are for high-protein dips to help you sneak some extra protein into your day and feel fuller for longer when you have a snack. This Smoked Salmon Dip is another great way to increase your intake of omega-3 fatty acids and could be the basis of a meal if you ate it with crostini and veggies. If you don't like the texture of cottage cheese, this dip is still worth trying because you'll be using a food processor to combine the ingredients, which smooths out the cottage cheese.

Yield: 8 servings

Ingredients

- 8 ounces (226 g) low-fat cottage cheese
- ¼ cup (70 g) plain nonfat Greek yogurt
- 2 tablespoons (27 g) mayonnaise
- ¼ teaspoon smoked paprika
- 1 tablespoon (15 ml) lemon juice
- 8 ounces (226 g) smoked salmon, roughly chopped
- 3 tablespoons (26 g) capers plus more for garnish
- 2 tablespoons (1 g) fresh dill, chopped, plus more for garnish
- 1 teaspoon lemon zest
- Salt and pepper to taste
- 2 medium scallions, chopped

You Will Need

- Food processor
- Measuring spoons
- ¼-cup measuring cup
- Spatula
- Knife
- Cutting board
- Bowl
- Beeswax or plastic wrap

Instructions

1. Add cottage cheese, Greek yogurt, mayonnaise, paprika, and lemon juice to a food processor and blend on high until smooth. You may need to stop the food processor to scrape the sides to make sure all the ingredients fully combine.

2. Add smoked salmon, capers, dill, and lemon zest to the food processor, and season with salt and pepper to taste. Pulse the food processor, pausing to scrape the sides if needed, until ingredients are just combined. The dip will be slightly chunky.

3. Transfer to a bowl. Cover the dip with beeswax or plastic wrap and chill for at least an hour. Taste and adjust seasonings as needed.

4. Store in the fridge and eat within 3 to 4 days of preparing. Do not leave out for longer than 3 hours (because of the dairy). Ideally, allow the dip to get to room temperature before eating. Serve with crudites (raw veggies of your choice) and crostini.

Elote Dip

I like to use the Elote seasoning from Trader Joe's in this recipe. If you don't have access to a TJ's, look for Elote or street corn seasoning at your local grocery store. You can also use this seasoning blend to make elote corn or in other dishes. This dip goes great with veggies and corn chips. Swap out the sour cream for Greek yogurt to make it higher in protein.

Yield: 6 servings

Ingredients

- 1 tablespoon (15 ml) olive oil
- 2 teaspoons minced garlic
- 1 [4-ounce (113 g)] can mild diced green chilies
- 1 [14.5-ounce (411 g)] can fiesta corn, rinsed and drained
- Salt and pepper, to taste
- ⅓ cup (76 g) mayonnaise
- ⅓ cup (93 g) plain nonfat Greek yogurt
- ⅓ cup (6 g) cilantro, chopped
- 1 tablespoon (15 ml) lime juice
- ¼ cup (32 g) crumbled queso fresco, divided
- 2 teaspoons elote seasoning
- Optional hot sauce, to taste

You Will Need

- Medium nonstick pan
- Measuring spoons
- Can opener
- Spatula
- Medium mixing bowl
- ¼-cup and ⅓-cup measuring cups
- Rubber spatula
- Beeswax or plastic wrap

Instructions

1. Add olive oil to a medium nonstick pan and place over medium-high heat. Add the garlic and green chilies and cook, stirring occasionally until fragrant, about seconds. Add the fiesta corn to the pan. Cook for 4 to 5 minutes, or until the corn is slightly browned, stirring occasionally. Season to taste with salt and pepper. Transfer the cooked corn mixture to a medium bowl and let cool for at least 10 minutes.

2. While the corn is cool, add the mayonnaise, Greek yogurt, cilantro, lime juice, 2 tablespoons (16 g) queso fresco, and elote seasoning to the bowl with the corn mixture. Use a rubber spatula to combine. Cover the bowl with beeswax or plastic wrap and refrigerate for at least 35 minutes. Garnish with remaining 2 tablespoons (16 g) queso fresco before serving.

3. Store in the fridge and eat within 3 to 4 days of preparing. Do not leave out for longer than 3 hours (because of the dairy).

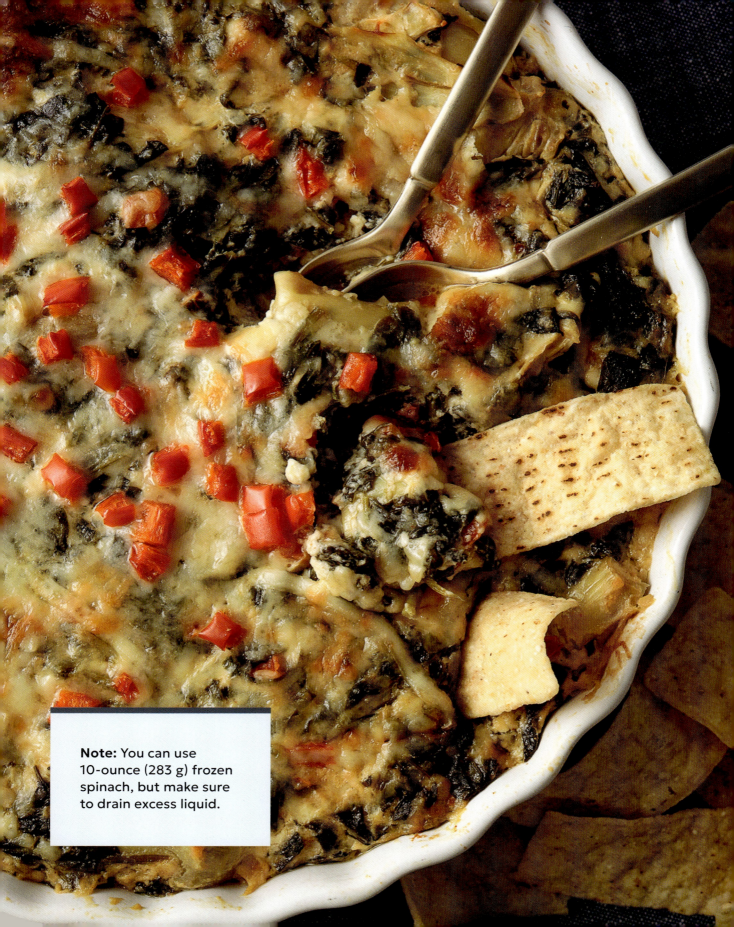

Note: You can use 10-ounce (283 g) frozen spinach, but make sure to drain excess liquid.

High-Protein Cheesy Spinach Dip

Spinach and artichoke dip is one of my favorite appetizers, and the red bell pepper adds a nice pop of color and crunch to this version. If using frozen spinach, thaw and drain the liquid to prevent the dip from getting watery. This dip is also great served on a flatbread.

Yield: 8 servings

Ingredients

- 1 tablespoon (15 ml) avocado oil
- ½ cup (94 g) finely chopped red bell pepper, plus 2 tablespoons (24 g) for topping
- 1 [1-pound (453 g)] package fresh spinach, roughly chopped (see note)
- 1 [14-ounce (397 g)] jar quartered artichoke hearts, drained
- ⅔ cup (151 g) low-fat cottage cheese
- 1 cup (245 g) plain nonfat Greek yogurt
- 1 cup (100 g) shredded Italian blend of cheese, divided
- ½ cup (50 g) shredded gruyere cheese, divided
- 2 teaspoons garlic powder
- 1 teaspoon onion powder
- ¼ teaspoon paprika
- Salt and pepper to taste

You Will Need

- 8" x 8" (20 x 20 cm) oven-safe baking dish
- Cooking spray
- Knife
- Cutting board
- Large nonstick pan
- Spatula
- Plastic mixing bowl
- ½-cup and 1-cup measuring cups
- Measuring spoons

Instructions

1. Preheat the oven to 400°F (204°C). Spray an 8" x 8" (20 x 20 cm) oven-safe baking dish with cooking spray and set aside.

2. In a large nonstick pan over medium heat, add avocado oil and red bell pepper. Cook until slightly softened, about 2 minutes. Add spinach to the pan, one handful at a time, stirring each time to help the spinach wilt and evaporate water, about 5 minutes.

3. Transfer the cooked spinach and pepper to a plastic mixing bowl. Add the rest of the ingredients to the bowl, except ¼ cup (25 g) of each of the shredded cheeses and 2 tablespoons (24 g) of chopped red bell pepper. Use a spatula to combine the ingredients until mixed well.

4. Pour the dip into the prepared baking dish. Top the mixture with the remaining shredded cheese and red bell pepper. Place the dish on the second from the top rack of the oven and bake for 30 minutes, baking until golden brown on top. To crisp up the top a little more, turn on the broiler on high and move the pan to the top rack. You will want to sit and watch it to prevent it from burning.

5. Remove the dish from the oven and let cool before serving. Serve with your favorite "dipables" such as tortilla chips or carrot sticks. Store in the fridge and eat within 3 to 4 days of preparing. Do not leave out for longer than 3 hours (because of the dairy).

French Onion Dip

French onion dip with some Lay's potato chips is a classic snack. This is a dip for one, so feel free to enjoy all of it.

Yield: 1 to 2 servings

Ingredients

- 1 cup (280 g) nonfat plain Greek yogurt
- 2 teaspoons mayonnaise
- 2 heaping tablespoons (8 g) dried minced onion
- ⅛ teaspoon garlic powder
- ⅛ teaspoon
- Worcestershire sauce
- ⅛ teaspoon salt

You Will Need

- Small bowl
- Spoon

Instructions

1. Add all of the ingredients to a small bowl and stir to combine. Cover the bowl with plastic wrap or beeswax for 10 minutes or until the dried onions are moistened.

2. Store in the fridge and eat within 3 to 4 days of preparing. Do not leave out for longer than 3 hours (because of the dairy). Serve with your favorite potato chips and/or veggies. Enjoy!

Omega-3 Rich Trail Mix

The nuts in this trail mix provide lots of omega-3s and minerals that are important for ADHD brains. I recommend using unsalted or lightly salted nuts if you need to be mindful of your sodium intake. Pro-tip: I keep my nuts in the freezer because it keeps them super fresh, and nuts are expensive.

Yield: 12 servings

Ingredients

- ½ cup (62 g) lightly salted shelled pistachios
- ½ cup (64 g) walnuts
- ½ cup (57 g) cashews
- ½ cup (72 g) pumpkin seeds
- ½ cup (80 g) dark chocolate chips
- ½ cup (61 g) dried cherries

You Will Need

- ½-cup measuring cup
- Medium mixing bowl

Instructions

1. Combine all the ingredients in a medium bowl and enjoy!

2. Store in an airtight container in a cool, dark place for up to 6 months. If stored in the freezer, this mix can last up to 2 years.

Resources

Books

Intuitive Eating by Evelyn Tribole and Elyse Resch

Anti-Diet: Reclaim Your Time, Money, Well-Being, and Happiness Through Intuitive Eating by Christy Harrison

The Wellness Trap: Break Free from Diet Culture, Disinformation, and Dubious Diagnoses, and Find Your True Well-Being by Christy Harrison

Fearing the Black Body: Racial Origins of Fat Phobia by Sabrina Strings

Gentle Nutrition by Rachael Hartley

Activate Your ADHD Potential: A 12-Step Journey from Chaos to Confidence for Adults With ADHD by Brooke Schnittman & Dr. Sharon Seline

ADHD 2.0 by Dr. Edward Hallowell & Dr. John Ratey

How to ADHD: An Insider's Guide to Working with Your Brain (Not Against It) by Jessica McCabe

Extra Focus: The Quick Start Guide to ADHD by Jesse Anderson

A Radical Guide for Women with ADHD by Sari Solden & Michelle Frank

ADHD for Smart Ass Women: How to Fall in Love with Your Neurodivergent Brain by Tracy Otsuka

How to Keep House While Drowning by KC Davis

The Neurodivergent Friendly Workbook for DBT Skills by Sonny Jane Wise

"You Just Need to Lose Weight" and 19 Other Myths About Fat People by Aubrey Gordon

The Body Is Not an Apology: The Radical Power of Self-Love by Sonya Renee Taylor

Podcasts

ADHD

I Have ADHD Podcast

Divergent Conversations

Adulting with ADHD

ADHD for Smart Ass Women

Women & ADHD

The ADHD Women's Wellbeing Podcast

ADHD Chatter Podcast

Successful with ADHD

ADHD rewired with Eric Trivers

Food & Body Image

Food Psych with Christy Harrison

Maintenance Phase

Body Kindness

Intuitive Bites Podcast

Diabetes Digital

Body Grievers Club Podcast

The Full Plate Podcast

Don't Salt My Game

Life After Diets

Dietitians Unplugged

Unbiased Science Podcast

The Nutrition Science Podcast

Websites

Intuitiveeating.org/studies/

Asdah.org

Howtoadhd.com

Understood.org

Add.org

Chadd.org

Therapyden.com

Ndtherapists.com

Inclusivetherapists.com

Social Media

ADHD Accounts

@coachingwithbrooke

@livedexperienceeducator

@authenticallyadhd

@currentadhdcoaching

@the_mini_adhd_coach

@adhdwithjennafree

@i.have.adhd.podcast

@haley.honeyman

@dt.perry

@theadhdcycle

@neurospicycounseling

@learning.compass

@hummingbird_adhd

@adhd_empower-
ment_coaching

@adhdjesse

@divergentcoachkelly

Dietitians, Therapists, and More

@adhd.nutritionist

@drcolleenreichmann

@theshirarose

@bodyimage.therapist

@bodyimagewithbri

@feelgooddietitian

@streetsmart.rd

@alissarumseyrd

@your.latina.nutritionist

@thenutritiontea

@thenutritionjunky

@eatingwithadhd

@chr1styharrison

@iamchrissyking

@v_solesmith

@kids.eat.in.color

@kid.food.explorers

@arfid.dietitian

@edadhd_therapist

@rds.neurodiversity

@the_adhd_rd

@nin.binge.adhd.nutrition

@pcos.nutritionist

@the.bloodsugar.nutritionist

@t1d.nutritionist

@prediabetes.nutrition

@healthyphit

@fork.diet.culture

@strugglecare

@colleenmwerner

@rachaelhartleyrd

@margos_wholebodynutrition

Acknowledgments

Writing a book as an ADHDer while also dealing with challenging circumstances in my personal life and running my virtual private practice was as challenging and rewarding as it sounds. This book would not exist without support from my publisher, family, friends, clients, and the online ADHD community. To all of the ADHDers I've had the opportunity to support as clients and interact with on social media: Thank you for sharing your experiences and challenging me to learn and grow into a better dietitian.

To my family and friends: Thank you for the emotional support and letting me write at your house when my upstairs neighbors were too loud. I want to thank my publishing team at The Quarto Group for helping me through every step of the writing and publishing process as a first-time author. Special thanks to Hilary for your patience and words of encouragement when I doubted myself; Chrystle, for helping edit the manuscript and hit the word count; Wendi, for your amazing photography skills; Mattie and Abby, for making my vision for the cover and book come to life.

About the Author

Rebecca King is a Registered Dietitian Nutritionist and Certified Intuitive Eating Counselor from Charlotte, North Carolina. She holds a bachelor of science in public health with a minor in women's studies from the University of South Carolina and a master of science in human nutrition from Winthrop University. She also completed her dietetic internship through Winthrop University and did the majority of her dietetic internship rotations at the VA Dorn Hospital in Columbia, South Carolina.

Rebecca is an adult with ADHD who struggled for years with disordered eating and chronic dieting. It wasn't until she discovered Intuitive Eating in graduate school that she was able to overcome binge eating and find food freedom.

Becca's first job as a dietitian was in a weight loss clinic. After seeing firsthand how much traditional dieting harmed her patients' relationships with food and being asked to provide weight loss advice to a bulimic patient, Rebecca decided she needed to do something different. After reflecting on her Intuitive Eating journey and working with other clients with ADHD, Rebecca saw a huge need for nutrition support for adults with ADHD. In July 2020, Rebecca founded ADHD Nutritionist LLC to help other ADHDers work with their brains so they can eat in a way that makes them feel their best mentally and physically. Her virtual private practice supports adults and teens with ADHD, who struggle with binge eating, chronic dieting, and body image issues, heal their relationship with food and find food freedom.

In her virtual private practice, Rebecca uses the Principles of Intuitive Eating and a weight-inclusive approach to nutrition. Rebecca has worked with over 200 clients in her small group coaching program or as private clients. Rebecca's popular Instagram page, The ADHD Nutritionist, is the #1 page for content relating to ADHD and food. Started in 2020, the page has grown to over 207k followers in four years and continues to attract new fans every day. Rebecca also maintains a busy podcast schedule, having been a guest on some of the biggest podcasts relating to ADHD, including the *I Have ADHD Podcast*, *ADHD for Bad Ass Women*, and *Adulting with ADHD Podcast*.

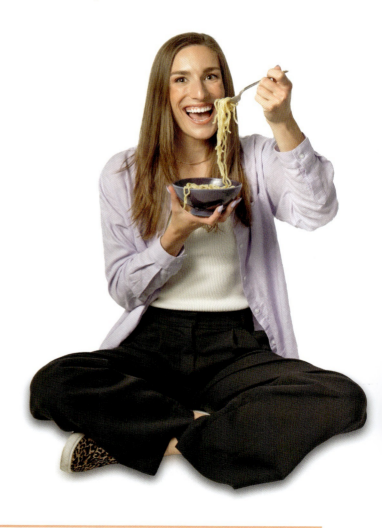

Index

A

ableism, 20, 127
AI, meal planning and, 113
air-foods, 43–44
air-fryer meals
    air fryers, 123
    Cheesy Chicken Nachos, 163
    Chicken Tender Wrap, 161
    Loaded Veggie Salad with Grilled Chicken, 165
    Shrimp Tostadas, 162
    Teriyaki Salmon Burgers, 166
alarms, 54
anti-fat bias, 20
apps
    Calm, 46
    doomscrolling prevention with, 79
    Headspace Meditation, 46
    Insight Timer, 46
    The Mindfulness App, 46
    grocery shopping and, 115
Atkins diet, 84
automation, 55, 68, 113
avoidant/restrictive food intake disorder (ARFID), 20

B

Barkley, Russell, 50
beige foods, 57
binge eating
    ADHD association with, 20
    ancestors and, 30
    brain hunger and, 38
    carbs and, 84
    control and, 40
    disordered eating and, 19
    dopamine and, 13, 71, 72, 73, 74
    emotional regulation and, 15, 37, 60–61
    hyperfocus and, 50
    Intuitive Eaters and, 17, 24
    medications and, 15, 56
    patterns and, 51, 55
    restricted eating and, 25
    time blindness and, 50
    triggers, 37, 67
    urge surfing and, 67
Binge/Restrictor avatar, 16, 30, 48–49
biological hunger, 35
blenders, 123
blood sugar, 24, 30, 50, 92, 93, 94, 95
body check-ins, 46
body doubling, 54
body scans, 46
brain hunger, 37–38, 74
breakfast
    Apple Cinnamon Overnight Oats, 129
    Avocado Toast with Fried Egg, 132
    Breakfast Tacos, 133
    Chunky Monkey Overnight Oats, 129
    consistency and, 55
    Egg Bites, 135
    Ham and Cheese Egg Bites, 135
    High-Protein Pancakes with Berries, 136
    Mixed Berry Chia Pudding, 130
    Overnight Oats, 129
    PB&J Overnight Oats, 129
    Spinach and Feta Egg Bites, 135
    Veggie-Packed Egg Bites, 135
Brown, Thomas E., 13
bulimia, 20, 71
B vitamins, 103

C

calorie requirements, 98
camouflaging. See masking
carbs, 94
check-ins, 46
chronic conditions, 26
classic recipes
    Cheeseburger Casserole, 178
    Chicken and Broccoli Mac and Cheese, 174
    Muffin Pan Chicken Pot Pies, 176
    Ramen Glow-up, 173
    Sausage and Veggie Pasta, 175
Clean-Plate Club, 42–43
cleanup
    anti-fatigue mats, 126
    aprons, 126
    bare minimums, 124
    companionship and, 125
    delegation, 125, 127
    dishes, 125
    dish soap, 126
    expectations, 124
    headphones for, 126
    kids and, 127
    music for, 126
    Reset Day, 124–125
    rubber gloves, 126
    strategies, 124–125
    struggling with, 127
    systems for, 125
    timers, 126
    tools for, 126
Community Supported Agriculture (CSA) boxes, 115
complex carbs, 94–95
consistency
    activity pairing and, 54
    alarms and, 54
    automation and, 55
    benefits of, 50–51
    Binge/Restrictor types and, 48–49
    blood sugar and, 50
    body doubling, 54
    breakfast and, 55
    dopamine and, 73
    establishing, 51–57
    "fed is best" mindset, 53
    Grazers and, 48, 49
    intention and, 50–51
    interoception and, 49
    meal patterns, 51–52
    medications and, 49, 56–57
    mood and, 50
    structure and, 49
    support for, 55
    time management and, 53
    visual cues for, 54
cooking strategies, 122–123
cravings
    emotional intensity of, 60
    honoring, 24, 27, 44

hunger and, 35, 38
L-tyrosine and, 100
novelty, 76
restriction and, 73
sugar cravings, 94

D

dance, 46
DASH (Dietary Approaches to Stop Hypertension), 86
Davis, KC, 124
Day-of Meal Planning, 112
diets
    Atkins diet, 84
    DASH (Dietary Approaches to Stop Hypertension), 86
    diet culture, 18, 23, 24
    eating patterns and, 85
    Feingold Diet, 83
    Few Foods Diet, 83
    gluten-free diet, 84
    ketogenic diet, 84
    Mediterranean diet, 85–86
    rigidity of, 22, 25
    social messaging and, 23
    as treatment strategy, 82
disordered eating, 19–20
dopamine
    consistency and, 73
    craving comprehension, 74
    Dopamenu, 76–80
    eating disorders and, 71
    food connection, 13, 71
    function of, 70
    hunger and, 73
    maximized stimulation, 74
    medications and, 72
    restriction and, 73
    snacks for, 80
    sources of, 70
    stimming, 71
    stimulation eating, 72, 74, 75
DSM-5 manual, 15, 59

E

eating disorders (ED). See specific disorders
eating patterns, 85
emotional eating
    binge eating and, 60–61
    boundaries for, 67
    cravings and, 60
    dieting and, 58, 60
    dysregulation of, 58, 59–61
    emotion identification, 62–64
    feelings compared to, 58
    Feelings Thermometer, 62–64, 65
    food as regulation of, 59–60
    hunger and, 37, 62
    interoception and, 61–64
    masking and, 62
    reflection and, 69
    restriction and, 60
    self-care checklist, 68–69
    self-care support, 69
    self-regulation toolkit, 66
    sensory safe spaces, 66
    strategies for, 64, 65
    support for, 69
    therapy and, 60
    toolkit for, 65–66
    triggers, 61
    urge surfing, 67
emotional regulation, 15
executive function (EF), 13, 14

F

fat-phobia, 23
fats, 97
"fed is best" mindset, 53
Feelings Thermometer, 62–64
Feingold Diet, 83
Few Foods Diet, 83
fiber, 95
fish oil, 103
Folate (B9), 103
food labels, 90, 92
food prep
    common barriers to, 121
    mise en place, 122
    recipe handling, 121
    selective meal prep, 121
    shortcuts for, 122
    task order, 121
freezer organization, 119
fullness
    air-foods, 43–44
    barriers to, 42
    boundary flexibility, 43
    Clean-Plate Club, 42–80
    companions and, 43
    emergence of, 45
    hunger/fullness scale, 45
    macronutrients and, 43
    restriction and, 43
    satisfaction and, 44
    sensory inputs and, 42, 45
    signs of, 40, 41
    snacking and, 42
    three-bite check-in, 42
    volume foods, 43

G

gentle nutrition
    environment and, 90–91
    incorporating, 89–90
    MyPlate guidelines, 93
    nutrient-dense foods, 90
    overcomplication and, 91
    saturated fats, 91
    sodium intake, 92
    sugar intake, 92–93
    unsaturated fats, 91
gluten-free diet, 84
Grazer avatar, 16, 48, 49
grocery shopping
    apps for, 115
    bulk buying, 117
    Community Supported Agriculture (CSA) boxes, 115
    delivery orders, 116
    noise-cancelling headphones for, 117
    peak hours, 116
    pickup orders, 116
    primary grocery stores, 116
    sensory-friendly hours, 116
    shopping lists, 115
    small grocery stores, 116–117
    strategies for, 116–117
    support for, 117

H

Hallowell, Edward, 47
Harrison, Christy, 23
headphones, 42, 117, 126
hunger
    barriers to, 39
    biological hunger, 35
    brain hunger, 37–38, 74
    chronic restriction, 39
    dieting and, 39
    dopamine and, 73
    emotional hunger, 37
    emotion and, 62
    hunger/fullness scale, 45
    interoception and, 74
    medications and, 35
    mindset and, 39
    physical hunger, 35
    practical hunger, 36–37
    primal hunger, 36
    rebound hunger, 36
    sickness and, 39
    signs of, 36, 37, 38
    stress and, 39
    taste hunger, 38
    types of, 35–38
hyposensitivities/hypersensitivities, 87

I

InstantPots, 123
intention, 35, 50–51
interoception
    body check-ins, 46
    body scans and, 46
    consistency and, 49
    definition of, 34
    emotional eating and, 61–64
    hunger and, 74
    medications and, 49
    meditation and, 46
    mindfulness and, 46
    somatic exercises and, 46
    support for, 46
Intuitive Eating (IE)
    avatar, 17
    benefits, 24
    chronic conditions and, 26, 30
    definition of, 24
    effectiveness, 22–23
    flexibility, 22
    myths, 29–31
    principles, 25–29
    structure, 30
    support for, 23
iron, 102

K

ketogenic diet, 84
"kid" foods, 57
kitchen organization
    freezer organization, 119
    fruit storage tips, 120
    organization tools, 118
    pantry organization, 118
    professionals for, 120
    refrigerator organization, 119
    tips for, 118
    veggie storage tips, 120

L

L-tyrosine, 100

M

macronutrients
    calorie requirements, 98
    carbs, 94–95
    complex carbs, 94–95
    fats, 97
    fiber, 95
    fullness and, 43
    monounsaturated fats, 98
    polyunsaturated fats (PUFAs), 98
    protein, 96
    saturated fats, 97–98
    simple carbs, 94–95
    unsaturated fats, 97
magnesium, 101
Mahler, Kelly, 46
masking, 62
Maybin, Moira, 79
meal kit services, 113–114
meal patterns, 51–52
meal planning
    9–1–1 plan, 114
    AI for, 113
    automating and, 113
    challenges, 107
    Day-of Meal Planning, 112
    meal evaluation, 109
    meal kit services, 113–114
    "Pick Three" meal planning, 112
    real-life examples, 110–112
    snacks, 109
    strategies for, 107–108
    time for, 108
medications
    consistency and, 49, 56–57
    dopamine and, 72
    food tolerance alternatives, 56–57
    hunger and, 15, 35
    interoception and, 49
    stimulants, 15, 56, 99, 100
meditation, 46
Mediterranean diet, 85–86
mindfulness, 46
mise en place, 122
monounsaturated fats, 98
multivitamins, 99
music, 42, 63, 64, 123, 126
MyPlate guidelines, 85, 93, 94, 95

N

no-heat and handheld meals
    Buffalo Chicken Wrap, 146
    Build Your Own ADHD Charcuterie Plate or Board, 143–144
    Chicken Gyro Wrap, 141
    Italian Pasta Salad, 147
    Walking "Tacos," 142
noise-cancelling headphones, 117
nootropics, 100–101
nutrient-dense liquids, 56–57

O

one-pot or one-pan meals
    Mediterranean Meatballs and Chickpea Orzo, 152
    Salmon Sheet Pan with Roasted Veggies and Potatoes, 150
    Sheet Pan Gnocchi and Veggies, 160

Six-Ingredient Chicken and Veggie Stir-Fry, 156
Southwestern Quinoa Salad, 149
Spicy Pickle Flatbread, 153
Steak or Shrimp Fajita Bowl, 155
Teriyaki Tuna Bowl, 159
organization. *See* kitchen organization
overwhelm
    cleanup, 124–127
    cooking, 122–123
    food prep, 121–122
    grocery shopping, 115–117
    kitchen organization, 117–120
    meal planning, 107–114

P

pantry organization, 118
Perfectionist avatar, 16
physical hunger, 35
"Pick Three" meal planning, 112
"picky eating," 17, 86, 88
polyunsaturated fats (PUFAs), 98
practical hunger, 36–37
primal hunger, 36
probiotics, 84
processed foods, 57

R

ready-to-eat foods, 57
rebound hunger, 36
reflection, 69
refrigerator organization, 119
Resch, Elyse, 24, 34
Riboflavin (B2), 103
rice cookers, 123

S

saturated fats, 91, 97–98
Selective Eater avatar, 17
self-care checklist, 68–69
senses
    charcuterie and, 143
    cleaning and, 124, 126
    grocery stores and, 115, 116, 117
    inputs, 42
    preferences, 26, 27, 42, 57, 113
    protein and, 96
    safe foods list, 89
    safe spaces, 66
    sensitivities, 17, 23, 81, 86–89
    sensory specific satiety, 45
serotonin, 13
shopping. *See* grocery shopping
simple carbs, 94–95
smoothies
    Berry Blast Smoothie, 137
    Cold Brew Smoothie, 139
    Strawberry Peanut Butter Smoothie, 138
    Tropical Paradise Smoothie, 138
snacks
    Elote Dip, 181
    Energy Balls, 179
    French Onion Dip, 184
    fullness and, 42
    High-Protein Cheesy Spinach Dip, 183
    "Kitchen Sink" Balls, 179
    meal planning and, 109
    Omega-3 Rich Trail Mix, 185
    Peanut Butter Dark Chocolate Balls, 179
    Smoked Salmon Dip, 180

    Strawberry Shortcake Balls, 179
sodium, 92
somatic exercises, 46
stimming, 71
stimulation eating, 74, 75
St. John's Wort, 100
storage. *See* kitchen organization
sugar intake, 86, 92–93
supplements
    B vitamins, 103
    fish oil, 103
    Folate (B9), 103
    iron, 102
    L-tyrosine, 100
    magnesium, 101
    multivitamins, 99
    nootropics, 100–101
    pros and cons, 99–100
    Riboflavin (B2), 103
    St. John's Wort, 100
    vitamin C, 102
    zinc, 101
support
    for consistency, 55
    for emotional eating, 69
    for grocery shopping, 117
    for interoception, 46
    for Intuitive Eating (IE), 23

T

tai chi, 46
Takeout Queens or Kings avatars, 16–17
taste hunger, 38
therapy, 20, 23, 30, 46, 60
three-bite check-in, 42
time management
    meal planning and, 108
    regular eating and, 53
    takeout and, 16
Tribole, Evelyn, 24, 34
triggers
    binge eating, 37
    boundaries for, 67
    eating disorders, 19, 37
    emotional eating, 37, 61, 67

U

unsaturated fats, 91, 97
urge surfing, 67

V

veggie-focused recipes
    Falafel Hummus Platter, 169
    Greek-Style Lentil Salad, 171
    Instant Pot Vegetarian Chili, 167
    Kitchen Sink Veggie Soup, 168
vitamin B, 103
vitamin C, 102
volume foods, 43

W

Wise, Sonny Jane, 66

Y

yoga, 46

Z

zinc, 101